For Sheila

Beyond the Melody

ISBN 978-0-9837768-9-5

Published in the United States by Yesteryear Publishing.

Books are available at **www.amazon.com** as well as through the author or publisher:

Yesteryear Publishing
P.O. Box 311
Hummelstown, PA 17036

www.yesteryearpublishing.com
yesteryearpublishing@gmail.com
(717) 566-8655

Beyond the Melody is unlike anything you have read before. It is a fitting tribute to two women of great substance who experienced an extraordinary journey and a friendship that most of us can only wish for.

Combining households was the easy part in light of what they later faced through a labyrinth of medical facilities, personnel, specialists, and, finally, hospice when Sheila resolutely faced her terminal illness. Nancy kept their many friends informed through beautifully crafted emails that were positive in their message while honest in the facts—not an easy task.

Seven years following the loss of Sheila, Nancy decided to memorialize this friendship by telling the story behind the emails. The result is riveting. The author's ability to inject humor into the daily travails of the journey allows the reader to identify with—and perhaps prepare for—this all too human and somewhat inevitable experience many may face.

Beyond the Melody

Table of Contents

Author's Notes

My life of sixty-plus years has been a blessed one. I have a loving family, good health, enriching friends, a sustaining and motivating church community, a sense of accomplishment in retirement from a meaningful career, and a pension that helps pay the bills for me and the cat. One period of my adult life was especially happy; during the time when Sheila Zinn was my friend. I knew her for seventeen years. We lived together for twelve of those years until she died in 2008.

During the final six months of Sheila's life when she was battling her illness in the hospital and at home, I corresponded with her friends and family via e-mail to keep them updated on her condition. Several weeks after her death, it occurred to me that those e-mails had captured a story I never anticipated nor envisioned myself able to endure if someone had outlined it before it began.

I was not able to access the "sent e-mail" file in our computer, so I asked the recipients to send these emails back to me, if anyone had retained them. Two people had all of them and kindly complied with my request. I had no plans for those e-mails. I just knew that I wanted them. I think it felt like hanging on to Sheila somehow during those initial dark summer days of dealing with the pain of her death.

Months later, the e-mails came to mind as I was in our office cleaning out some things. I remember thinking that there was so much more to the story of our last six months together than I had written in those e-mails. The true picture of our friendship and

Sheila's final months was not fully captured. "Maybe I should write more, fill in the blanks around those e-mails," I thought to myself. A short while later, I tried to do it.

I copied the texts into a Word document to begin a manuscript. But I could not write. Nothing came to me and I cried as I thought about how 2008 had been for Sheila and me. So I stopped trying. I didn't even re-read my own correspondence to those faithful friends. I thought that was the end of it. I even considered deleting the e-mails and the Word document. But something made me keep them.

During the next seven years, I felt "nudges" to do something with the treasure trove I had pasted into that Word document. Several times, I sat to write more and did not produce much. Once or twice, I did manage to make a few brief notes about what I remembered was happening in our lives outside of Sheila's illness. But my manuscript really contained little other than the copied e-mails. The nudges kept me from deleting them.

I have learned through my lifetime that responding to nudges, which I believe are of the spirit of God, leads me to interesting (sometimes unusual or scary) decisions. I try to do what I'm nudged to do because I believe it is part of living a faithful life, a priority for me. I finally felt ready to respond when, seven years after her death, several of my new friends in my new hometown asked about Sheila when I mentioned her. I occasionally spoke about my Ohio friend to my Pennsylvania friends and they were caring and attentive enough to want to know more.

This time, when I sat to write, I did not cry (at least initially), and I found that the story unfolded in my mind relatively easily. It's almost like it was given to me. I don't usually have a good memory, but re-reading those e-mails brought so many things to me quite clearly. I worked chronologically and just wrote the story down as I remembered it. I worked on it for several months, nearly every day. I kept the Kleenex box handy because it was not easy to re-live Sheila's final days and the immediate months thereafter.

When I finished the story, I didn't know what to do next. So I didn't do anything. I felt satisfied that I had completed the work, but I did not read it. I had done some light editing as I went and I did a spell check when I was finished, but that was the extent of my effort. I was emotionally spent and comfortable with my "do nothing" plan.

After a few weeks, I realized that if I wanted my manuscript to be a means by which my new friends could get to know Sheila, I would have to share it with them. I wasn't even sure, though, that what I had written would be understood or interesting to anyone else. I decided that I had to find someone who would read the manuscript and provide feedback. I thought of a person in my new church who is kind-hearted, well-read, a poet, and an editor. I thought she might agree to help me by reading and reacting. She generously took time to do just that and assured me that the story was funny and revealing. She suggested the names of others who she thought would very much want to read it. I felt tentative and uneasy.

Encouraged by the first reader, I invited several other friends, two of whom are published authors, to read and provide candid feedback. In all cases, my Pennsylvania friends validated the work and encouraged me to make the story available to others. Even with this reinforcement, I was hesitant, surprised by their enthusiasm for publishing. I became unsure about revealing more details about my twelve years with Sheila, and I began to realize the extent to which our lives could be exposed to criticism or judgment. I was getting into very uncomfortable territory, as happens when God nudges.

I had to find a way to be confident in next steps, since the enthusiastic feedback I was receiving from my friends was far beyond what I ever envisioned. I decided to walk a labyrinth. I had done so once previously and, despite skepticism, found it to be a very meaningful experience. I located a labyrinth on the grounds of a Lancaster County church, confirmed that it is open to the public, and visited on a beautiful summer afternoon. I entered the path after resting and clearing my mind, asking the question, "What now for my manuscript?"

I received two very clear messages: use the people and share the story. I felt like I was already using the people in my life to help me. The message seemed to be: "These people have been given to you. They know what they are talking about. They are uniquely talented and care about you. They will continue to help you. Use them."

During that walk, I was also reminded that Sheila's very presence in my life was a great gift. The things we experienced together were unique, as is true for any two people who share life's experiences. That I could write something readable about that and have it be well received was a continuation of the gift. I resolved to forge ahead, believing that I should trust God's nudges once again and share the story.

I next shared the manuscript with three friends who knew and loved Sheila. Every reader prior to this had known only me; these three additional readers had been recipients of the e-mails and were part of the story. I needed their feedback before I could be completely comfortable escalating my work to become a project to publish a book. These friends were also affirming and encouraging. I was now committed, but the path forward was still uncertain. There was so much to learn.

I had the perfect teacher. A long-time friend, school administrator, English teacher, college professor, writer, and editor had been one of the first readers of my manuscript. She agreed to shepherd me through the work necessary to publish a book. I trusted her completely and felt confident that we could work well together. Thus began our process of editing, finding a suitable title, and writing the additional components of a book beyond the manuscript itself.

Several readers of the book in its early crude form encouraged me to categorize it according to its theme. "Decide what it's about, Nancy, so you can figure out how to market it when you publish it. It will help you to understand how it may appeal to potential readers." I decided to ignore that counsel because I don't know what this book is about. The first readers say it's about friendship, terminal illness, devotion, grief, cohabitation, love, hospice care, with some "comic relief" woven through.

The only sure thing I know is that this is the story of Sheila and me. I wrote it as accurately and truthfully as I could. I am not a writer. I have never been motivated to write a book about anything. I am not motivated to market or sell this story. I'm publishing it because I feel led to do so and will, as Sheila once said; " … trust God for the outcome." I hope you will find meaning for yourself as you read. If you do, you will have discovered what it's about.

Prelude

The phone rang in my office just before eleven in the morning on January 2, 2008. I could see from the display that it was Sheila, my housemate of twelve years and a very infrequent caller. She had been ill with significant digestive problems during the entire month of December and I was very worried about her. She was awaiting an appointment with a gastroenterologist, but progress was not expected until later in the week. I was puzzled, but not alarmed.

As it was the first work day of a new year, I was in the midst of plowing through an inbox loaded with e-mail, greeting everyone who had taken vacation over the holidays, and generally attempting to get my head back into doing my job providing leadership for a customer service team that was at the height of a busy season. I answered the phone not knowing what to expect.

"I'm sorry to bother you, but I was in the doctor's office for my foot and on the way out, the nurse told me that they heard from the gastroenterologist. He suggested that I come to the ER and have him paged. This has gone on too long. He said this will be the quickest way for me to see him. Can you come home and take me?"

I was about to go to a two-hour meeting that I had arranged with a group of people whose schedules made them nearly impossible to convene. I did not want to reschedule the meeting, especially on five minutes notice. But I knew how eager Sheila was to receive treatment. We always supported each other fully, especially in times of need. My mind was rapidly thinking through options so I could make a suggestion that would work for both of us.

Finally, I said, "Sheila, I think we have two choices." I explained the circumstances of my imminent business obligation. "I would like to go to this meeting. I can come home after one o'clock and take you or you can get there sooner if we think of someone else who could give you a ride. What would you like to do?"

Without hesitation, Sheila declared that she did not want to wait. We conferred about people who could provide ER taxi service on short notice in the middle of a January weekday and came up with a list of possibilities.

At the conclusion of this dialogue, I asked her if she had finished making the e-mail distribution list that we had discussed when we were anticipating her treatment, which we expected to require hospitalization. Sheila's network of friends and family was extensive. I had implored her to prepare the list so I could keep everyone updated while she received treatment. She promised to finish the list before going to the hospital.

Ever the take-charge sort, Sheila then ushered me off to my meeting with a promise that she would call back and leave a message in my voice mail to confirm that a driver had been located. I told her I would meet her at the hospital later in the afternoon as soon as I could get away from the office. Little did I know that we were about to begin a journey that would change my life.

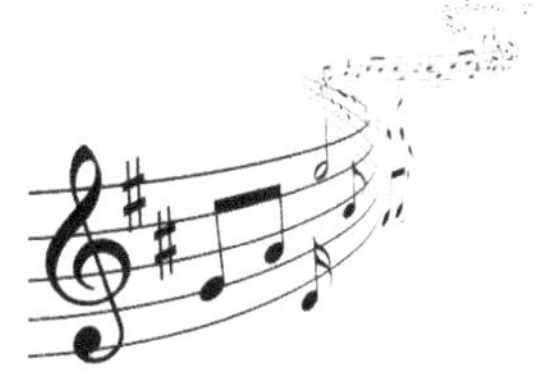

Unison and Harmony

History

Sheila and I met in church in 1991. I was a transplant from central Pennsylvania to central Ohio because of a job promotion. I knew almost no one in the area, but was confident that making the move was what I was led to do. Shortly after settling in Grove City, Ohio, I began church shopping and ultimately selected the smaller of the two United Methodist churches in town because I thought I would get to know people sooner in a small congregation.

Sheila's husband, Allan, was the first person I met. Actually, he met me. I was giving myself a guided tour of the church education building when he approached and casually remarked about my experience ringing handbells. To my surprise, this was apparently common knowledge among several of the church members because of a letter sent by my former pastor to Grove City, alerting the local churches that I was coming to town. Allan was eager for us to meet because he was recruiting me to assist with the development of a new handbell choir in this little congregation. We spoke for a few brief moments, with my being highly noncommittal about helping him, before going our separate ways.

It was months later, after Allan's gentle and persuasive ways resulted in my becoming the new handbell director, that I met Sheila. She used to say that she recalled the exact moment. I don't. "You had a very firm handshake and looked me right in the eye when you introduced yourself. I liked that." I remembered only that Sheila and Allan were pillars of the church, involved in everything, and exceptionally likeable. I wanted to get to know both of them better.

Despite our busy schedules, we managed to build the foundation of a very pleasant friendship. Allan was in sales for a regional music company and Sheila was a music teacher in a local elementary school. The parents of three grown children, they had been college sweethearts and married for over thirty-five years when I began to know them. We occasionally got together for a meal or spent time in conversation after church. And they both helped me a great deal with the fledgling handbell choir. I'm not a musician, but I could ring bells and they were encouraging my efforts with the new group, much like parents rooting at a child's first independent endeavor.

Everything suddenly changed one autumn two years later. After months of discomfort from a persistent cough and inconclusive visits with doctors, Allan was diagnosed with advanced kidney cancer that had metastasized to his liver. The prognosis was grave, but my new friends were determined to put up a fight. They researched, consulted, prayed, and outlined a plan with the doctors. Allan had several surgeries, multiple treatments, and expert care at the Ohio State University Arthur James Cancer Hospital. But despite the best efforts of everyone, Allan died at home the following May. Sheila was his primary caregiver with the help of their children and the support of the local hospice organization.

Allan's death dealt a blow that rattled Sheila both physically and emotionally. I recall asking the pastor, "Who's helping her?" Our friendship was still new and our in-depth conversations scant, so I wasn't sure of Sheila's support network beyond the church people we had in common. The pastor's reply was immediate, "I think her children will be very attentive and Sheila's a strong woman. She'll be fine."

I didn't doubt that she would be fine, but I also thought that someone who had lost a spouse required support from friends in addition to the comfort her children could provide; after all, they had lost their father. I resolved to observe Sheila closely.

I developed a routine of calling her on the phone about once a week, just to see how she was doing and to determine if she needed to talk. Sheila seemed to welcome my efforts and spoke openly about the rigors of the grieving process. One day she mentioned that several people were insistently suggesting that it was time for her to pack up Allan's clothes and remove them from the house. "But I don't want to do that. I don't mind that they're here. Why do I have to rush into doing that?"

I think she sincerely wanted my perspective so I gave it to her. I told her to trust herself. "There is no proper way to do this. You have to do it your way. You will know when it's the right time to take on a task or go somewhere. And sometimes you will think you're ready and your experience will prove you wrong. There is no timetable for any of the things that must be done after a loved one dies. Anyone who tells you different is wrong. And anyone who tells you the pain goes away is wrong. It may not be as acute as time goes by, but it will not go away."

I really believed what I said based on prior experience being close to people who experienced the loss of loved ones. Sheila apparently heard a ring of truth to what I said because she began to call me. As time passed, we began to talk almost every day. I came to admire her for her "pluck," as my grandmother would describe it. She was open about her pain and the enormity of her grief, but she was determined to soldier on. She had attended a meeting of a hospice support group, but rejected future visits ("There were too many people looking backward. I want to look forward.") She also went to a local widows group because she thought she could help others, but ultimately bowed out ("I don't like the label 'widow.' It suggests that I'm weak and pitiful. I don't want to be weak and pitiful.")

As I began to know Sheila better, I became more comfortable approaching her and sharing things about myself. I am by nature an introvert, comfortable being alone, reticent, cautious with strangers, more tired than energized by parties, and prone to process thoughts before feelings. Sheila was quite the opposite. She experienced the world in terms of her feelings, invited everyone into her life, enjoyed the company of strangers and misfits ("I feel sorry for her/him"), and suffered when alone too long. We began to appreciate each other immeasurably.

Her bravery was impressive. She wrote letters to her children on Father's Day, within weeks of Allan's death. She told them why he was proud of them and what he especially loved about them. She told me she cried and cried and cried until she thought she could cry no more, but that she wanted to do it for them since she knew Father's Day would be hard for them.

Allan had been the choir director at church and Sheila a dedicated member. After the summer recess, the choir members convened in late August under new direction. The idea was to have an informal get-together to help the group move on without Allan and to help the new director become acclimated. I thought we were going to sing hymns and have refreshments. Sheila told me that she expected it to be a hard thing for her to do, but she wanted to participate because she liked singing in the choir, she enjoyed the people, and she did not want to give in to the pain.

That evening, I was seated behind Sheila, over her left shoulder. I was quite surprised when the new director, previously a member of the choir, pulled out the choir music we had been using during Allan's tenure and began to lead us through it. I could see that several of the songs were causing a tear or two for Sheila, but she remained collected and continued to sing. I was so impressed by her will to carry on.

But it all came to a halt when, implausibly to me, we were asked to sing "Shall We Gather at the River." I could see that Sheila had stopped singing and I couldn't stand seeing her struggle through this situation any longer. I tapped her on the shoulder and motioned for her to follow me out the door and up the steps. I led the way and turned around to face her as she traversed the final step. I opened my arms and invited her into a hug. She fell into my arms and sobbed.

I didn't say anything, just held on to her until we had to locate some Kleenex and she said, "That was more than I could take. I lived with that music and hearing it again was hard to do. Allan often played those songs on our piano. I'm glad this first time is over with. I think I'll do better next time. Thank you for getting me out of there." But she was determined to rejoin the group after collecting herself so nobody would be "overly sorry" for her and so the new director "wouldn't feel bad."

I learned to assess when Sheila was having a bad day and tried to be available to her during our evening conversations. I remember one evening in March when she had called early, in tears, but by the time I got home and found her message, she already had gone to a church meeting.

I decided that, in this case, distraction and laughter would be appropriate and met her in her driveway later that night with the newspaper version of the NCAA men's basketball brackets in my hand. I knew that Sheila was far from being a sports fan, but I wasn't able to come up with anything else after a long day at the office followed by a dinner meeting. I knew that anyone can complete a bracket.

For years my family has participated in the annual event with the winner owning bragging rights for the year. Sheila was very surprised to see me sitting in my car in her driveway, but she welcomed my visit and invited me in. We talked a bit about her painful week and then I introduced her to "bracketology." "Well," she asked, "how do you know who to pick?"

"Nobody knows, Sheila, but everyone tries. Some in the family think they know a lot about basketball and others have no idea. But there is no harm in trying."

I was surprised when she wanted to keep the paper to do some research before completing her entry, including a plan to better understand the concept of seeding in an athletic contest.

The following day, I was pleasantly surprised when Sheila called and informed me that she had completed her bracket and wanted me to look it over. I told her I would make no recommendations, but would review it if she wanted me to.

Her selections were indicative of her interests in the arts rather than athletics. "I chose Georgetown because my maiden name was George. I chose all of the Ohio schools because the local people should support those boys. I chose Gonzaga (to go to the final four, no less, unheard of in those days) because I liked the sound of that name." And so on.

From this silly exercise, I learned about Sheila's competitive side, which she denied ever existed. "I really don't care who wins," she insisted. But I found a copy of her completed bracket right beside her favorite chair for TV viewing with little red marks beside her successful selections. She was keeping score!

And to the amazement of everyone, Sheila was the champion that year, followed by my niece Elizabeth, who was four years old at the time. They clearly humbled all of us who prided ourselves on being knowledgeable basketball fans. They also did an excellent job of reminding us of their superiority in bracket selection at every opportunity thereafter.

Home ♫

Sheila and I soon fell into a routine of helping each other when either of us was involved in activities we preferred not to handle or when we just needed help because of time or lack of skill. She did not like yard work, so I helped her pull weeds and eradicate poison ivy from her yard. I didn't cook much, so she highly recommended various crock pot recipes and took great pride when I reported that everything turned out to be delicious.

When I went out of town, she fed the cats, watered the plants, and took in the mail at my house. I helped her shovel her very long driveway after a significant snow accumulation and she helped me select new wallpaper for my kitchen.

One time, after we had helped each other quite a bit over the course of several months, one of us said, "You know, this would be easier if we only had one house instead of racing back and forth for a mile and a half each time we help each other." And shortly thereafter, we began to consider the possibility of combining our households.

We talked about it kiddingly for a short while and then began to get serious. Sheila acknowledged that she did not like living alone. She had not really ever done so, having gone from her parents' home to college, then to marriage. I was somewhat weary of maintaining a household alone and living with the reality that, if anything got done around the house, it happened because I did it. There was nobody to help.

We agreed that we were compatible, enjoyed each other's company, and shared the values of faith, family, and service. I was concerned that, having lived alone for all of my adult life, I would not adjust well to living with someone. Sheila was quite sure we could work through anything that came up. And we began to talk about how we might actually combine households.

We agreed on financial independence, other than funds necessary to run the household, and we agreed that we wanted to be joint owners of whatever house we lived in. And we agreed that it would be smart to consult with an attorney to learn more about what would be involved and what issues we should think about as two unrelated people who might create a household together.

We both had attorneys who helped us with our wills and other legal matters. But we agreed that it would be best to seek out someone who would be independent and who might have experience in situations like this, something we were relatively sure neither of our attorneys had. We finally found someone with whom we met, but who provided very little in the way of suggestions or counsel. Next we located someone else, but that visit was equally unsatisfactory.

One thing that did come out of the discussions was a recommendation that we sell both of our houses and buy another one together. This approach would be most advantageous given the tax laws. We discussed that at length and discarded that counsel. Sheila's house was a wonderful five-bedroom, two-story on a large lot—and it was paid for, thanks to the hard work and prudent decisions that she and Allan had made along the way.

We agreed that the size of the house made it a perfect venue for what we had in mind, and the fact that both of us would not have to move made even more sense—but I did not want to feel like a tenant and wanted equity interest in my home.

Finally, Sheila consulted with her attorney about the possibility of selling half of her house, making us joint owners. During the course of that discussion when he agreed that she could sell half of the home if she wanted to, he suggested that we put the house and contents in a trust, of which we would be joint trustees. Sheila briefed me on that idea after her meeting with him and we liked it. So we began to discuss provisions of this trust, which Sheila's attorney drafted and my attorney reviewed.

After reviewing the legal documents, we agreed to combine our households and began to think about how we would tell people about our plans. We were both concerned about the perceptions of our families or friends and several other issues. I was concerned that we were making a move too soon after Allan's death and if I was being unfair to Sheila in agreeing to a move so quickly. She was concerned about my career plans and the possibility that I would decline future promotions that required relocation.

We talked and talked about the practical and emotional implications of what we were doing. But the driving factor in our decision to proceed was that we both believed that we could be better people if we were together than we would be if we were apart. Our friendship had become so significant for both of us that it was enriching our lives in ways we had not anticipated. We sincerely believed that we could contribute more and make a bigger difference in our worlds if we made a life together.

Shortly thereafter I listed my house for sale and we began the monumental task of sorting through two households full of accumulated belongings trying to figure out what to dispose of and what to keep. In Sheila's case, she was still housing some things from the teenage years of her children who had been out of the house for years. In my case, I had boxes in my basement that were never unpacked from four years prior when I had moved to Ohio. We decided that the logical thing to do was for each of us to identify which of our possessions were most precious so we could find a place for them in our home.

After hours of working through possessions, giving things away, moving small things to our house in the back of our cars, and selling my house, in November of 1996 the U-Haul truck and several friends appeared in my driveway and the final move began. It was an exciting day and a little bit overwhelming, but I had such a good feeling that it was the right decision and I was quite sure that Sheila felt the same way. It's hard to describe how committed we were to doing this for what seemed to be all the right reasons. Now that it was happening it was just a matter of doing the hard work to turn our plans into a reality. It was time for us to see if we really could be better people and better contributors because of making a life together.

Family

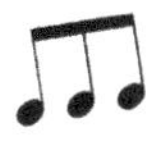

Sheila's parents had been in their sixty-fourth year of marriage when her father died, not long after I moved to Ohio. I never got to know him very well, but clearly remember something touching about her parents and their support for Sheila. She was still teaching music at the time and her annual spring concert was being held at the high school in the district where she taught. I wanted to see her in action so I got the details about the time and location and headed out for the event.

As I arrived, I could see Allan parking their van and walking toward the school entrance. He greeted me, but kept walking quickly toward the building, explaining that he had just dropped off his in-laws and wanted to catch up to them to ensure their safe transition to seats in the auditorium. Sheila's dad was leaning heavily on his cane, shuffling along toward the auditorium, while her mother took the arm Allan extended to help her. I remember thinking how touching it was to see that, no matter how old we become, good parents are interested in our activities.

Our families both included a history of teachers and teaching careers. Both fathers did additional work to supplement the family's income, Sheila's dad farming and my dad officiating at football and basketball games. Both of our mothers took time from their teaching careers to stay home with their children for a few years, then returned later to teach until retirement. Sheila was a music teacher and I had taught for several years before a career change.

Another trait we had in common was strong family ties and

support. Before I knew Sheila very well at all, I learned in church one Sunday that she had traveled to Alabama to be with her sister-in-law, Barbara, who was in hospice care. Her brother had no children and there were apparently no close relatives on the other side of the family, so Sheila went to lend support. She intended to stay there to help them until after her sister-in-law's death.

I remember thinking "What a generous thing to do. I'm not sure I would do that." I was impressed with Allan, too, who showed no signs of discontent or impatience with her absence as days turned into weeks. In fact, his sense of humor and gentle nature enabled him to play it up a bit. The congregation wanted to tend to him in Sheila's absence, so he was plied with food and entertainment of various sorts during this time.

Not too long after Barbara died and Sheila returned home, I remember her telling me how difficult it had been for her to watch the suffering of her sister-in-law and how grateful she was for the exceptional help from hospice care. "And," Sheila added, "I want to write my obituary. I have definite ideas about how I want it to be done. I must get to that soon."

A year following Barbara's death, Allan was diagnosed and Sheila again became care-giver for a family member. I remember her telling me that Allan had been reluctant to have hospice care, but Sheila's experience in Alabama had clearly informed her positive opinions on this service.

And, again, she mentioned her intent to write her obituary.

During Allan's illness, their children were present and attentive to both their mother and father, from what I could observe from a distance. After his death they continued to call their mother occasionally, but were not in constant communication. Her son Mark and his wife Tina, who lived about an hour away, came to visit almost every other week. Those Saturday evening times were good for Sheila, who spent the day preparing one of her tasty meals. In the fall, Buckeye football games were often on the television during the visits.

Our house was most tested by the invasions of my family from Pennsylvania during summer months. With some regularity, we had four extra adults and four children bunking in with us. My youngest brother, Bob, and his wife Lynn have four children. Lynn's sister lives in Indianapolis. It was common for them to make an annual trip with my parents in tow, stopping by our house on Friday evening for a Sheila meal and a game night. On Saturday, that family would travel on to Indiana while my folks stayed with us until the gang came back to pick them up for the return to Pennsylvania.

The kids loved Sheila's dog and Honey loved them. Blanche the cat was none too impressed by children, but the other cat, Ernie, was quite tolerant of excited little people petting him and inviting him to play. We took walks with the dog, made homemade ice cream and generally enjoyed each other's company.

When the kids and their parents learned about Sheila's interest and aptitude for music, it soon became standard practice for them to bring their instruments along for impromptu concerts. We had a violin, flute, and piano player in the bunch. They brought their music and Sheila made up accompaniment on the spot. For fledgling musicians, this was a big deal. And they had no idea how unusual it is for someone to have the gift that Sheila had to be able to do that.

I liked Sheila's mother, Mary, who was nearly ninety years old when Sheila and I made our home together. Sheila told me that her mother's only reservation was to wonder how two strong-willed women could keep disagreement out of the household. I'm not sure how she knew that I was strong-willed, but she certainly knew her daughter.

On one occasion when Sheila was away before I had moved in, I looked in on her mother. Mary said to me, "You know, Sheila has always been very high-spirited. She has a mind of her own." I don't know if that was intended to be a warning or a test.

I replied, "Yes, that is what I especially like about her." And that was the end of that.

Sheila was very attentive to her mother, especially after her father died in 1993. Sheila took her for groceries, to doctor appointments, to her hair appointments, and wherever else she needed to go. Since neither one was much of a sports fan, they even made a point of going Christmas shopping on the day of the Ohio State -Michigan football game because nobody was in the stores or the highways.

Because Mary did not drive and Sheila had retired from her teaching career, she was available to provide needed support for her mother, whose wit and mental capabilities were stellar, being fully engaged in life and interacting by phone and letter with her many friends and extended family. After the painful deaths of Clarence, Barbara, and Allan, things seemed to be settling down for Sheila and Mary. But not for long.

Sheila was traveling in Australia with her grandson, Joe. The previous summer she had taken her granddaughter Claire to France and Switzerland, her first trip after Allan died. Sheila loved to travel and feared that Allan's death would curtail her adventures. Upon hearing this, Claire said, "Grandma, I'll go with you." So they went to the place of Claire's choosing and this summer was Joe's turn.

Not long into their trip, I received a call at my office from Connie, Sheila's daughter, telling me that her grandmother had fractured her leg, was in the hospital, scheduled for surgery the next day. Sheila's brother Steve was on the way from Alabama and Connie wanted to know if he could stay at the house with me. Of course, I told her that would be fine and I asked for details about which hospital Mary was in and about her overall condition. Connie told me that Mary was holding up well and that they had all decided against calling Sheila to tell her this news because they didn't want her to cut short the trip with Joe. I didn't like that decision but didn't say anything. I needed time to think and to assess the situation more fully.

When I was able to leave the office, I went right to the hospital. During the twenty minute drive, I thought about how it would feel to be Sheila, who was close to her mother and who, I thought, would want to know that something had happened. I would have wanted to know. I had absolute confidence that Sheila would not do anything rash and I was confident that she would trust what I would tell her. So I was headed to gather information.

When I arrived at the hospital and found Mary's room, she was propped up in bed, alone, and looking pretty good. Her leg hurt only if she moved it, so, she explained, she tried not to move it. After general conversation about how she felt and what the surgeons had told her (yes, it was a bit risky to do surgery on a ninety-one year old diabetic lady, but they thought she would come through the procedure just fine), I asked her about informing Sheila.

Mary's reply assessed the situation, "If Sheila were here, she would be organizing everything and everyone and generally taking charge. It's good for my grandchildren to have to figure this out without her. I don't want her to feel like she has to come racing home. Everything will be fine. I don't want to ruin her trip with Joe. Now, you have to be warned about Stephen. I understand he's coming to stay at your house. He's sometimes petulant and difficult to get along with, so don't let him get to you."

"Mary, I think Sheila would want to know about this," I said. "I can persuade her that there is no need for her to come home. I can tell her that I've visited you and what your feelings are about her continuing the trip. I think she should know and I should be the one to tell her. It's not right to keep this news from her and for her to be surprised when she gets home and realizes that we kept it from her."

Mary considered my argument and saw my point of view. I did feel strongly that withholding the news of her mother's accident from Sheila was somehow dishonest. I had promised Sheila that I would not lie to her. This felt like a situation that called for me to honor that promise. I didn't think I needed to consult with the kids on this. I believed that this was among Mary, Sheila, and me. I was happy to have found Mary alone and capable of listening to my suggestion.

After imploring me to tell Sheila to continue her trip, and with my persuading her that I could do just that, Mary agreed that I should call Sheila to tell her about the situation. I spent the time on the drive home trying to figure out the time difference between eastern daylight saving time and Australia time—and contemplating what it would be like to have a house guest described by his own mother to be "petulant."

I figured out that if I called as soon as I got home, I might catch Sheila before they began their day's activities. It worked out that way. She listened to my assurances that the situation was not an emergency, her mother was adamant that she continue the trip, and I would call her to come home if I thought she needed to be here. She took the hospital phone number and details about her mother's room number and doctor's name, and promised that she would not make plans to cut the trip short. Mary came through the surgery without complications, the kids were faithful in attending to their grandmother, and I survived "petulant" Steve.

But Mary would never go home again. She did well after the procedure, but things got difficult during her rehabilitation process. Her heart was not strong enough to withstand the rigors of the physical therapy necessary for her to use the leg again. The doctors and therapist could never find the proper balance of effort and medication to enable her to regain the strength in her leg. She spent weeks in the rehab facility and, with no further progress expected, was moved to the nursing home division of the facility which had become her new home.

Sheila visited faithfully and Mary loved being a "test case" for the student nurses who did not usually have exposure to an elderly patient with a mind as sharp as Mary's. She told Sheila that it was important to her to serve in such a capacity. It gave her limited life meaning to be able to help the nursing students learn about eldercare.

Mary, however, finally became weary of her limitations and decided to decline further treatment for her heart condition and diabetes. She discussed her plans with Sheila and her doctor, who supported her completely. Sheila was pained, but realized that her quality of life had become significantly diminished and that her mother should be able to make decisions about the end of her life.

Mary signed the necessary documents regarding her decision, called the people she wanted to talk with before her death, organized visits with her grandchildren and great grandchildren for final conversations, and soon quietly slipped into an unconscious state.

I was watching Sheila closely to see how this was affecting her. She was distracted and a bit subdued, understandably, but very much supported her mother's decision. Steve came to visit and then went back to Alabama to await word from us about his mother's death.

I received a call at my office one afternoon from Sheila telling me that her mother was not expected to live through the coming night. I was surprised when she asked me to come to be with her at the nursing home. Her son Mark was already there, but she wanted me to come, too. I had not considered that I would be invited into this circumstance beyond supporting Sheila as best I could.

I left the office early with a sense of unease. I had never been present at someone's death before, so I did not know what to expect. But I decided that it didn't matter. Sheila needed me and I was going to be there. When I arrived, Sheila asked me to stay with her mother for a while so she and Mark could go to the end of the hall for coffee. "If anything changes, please come get us," she said and quietly moved out of the room and headed down the hall.

As I sat there, several members of the staff who had obviously been advised of Mary's declining condition came in to say their good-byes. They gently took her hand and spoke to her quietly, some thanking her for sharing her feelings and medical details with them. Some mentioned what a privilege it had been to help to take care of her. There were many tears shed over the impending death of this wonderful woman. I was impressed by their effort to come to see her, their sincere expression of gratitude, and their expression to her of goodbye and peace. It was extremely touching to see those people tending to one of their patients for the last time.

Soon, I noticed that Mary's breathing had become highly irregular, so I went down the hall to alert Sheila and Mark. Shortly after they came back into the room and when Sheila told her mother again that it was OK for her to go, Mary died. With a few tears leaking from her eyes, Sheila reached across her mother's bed, took my hand, and said, "We have just witnessed a high holy moment."

Several days after her mother's funeral service, Sheila again said to me "I must take time to write my obituary. I have definite ideas about how I want my obituary to be written, so I'm going to do it myself." This obituary writing was really something with her, I could see.

Animals

Sheila and I were both pet owners when we combined our households. She had a dog and two cats, one of which lived exclusively in her basement because of a colossal inability to get along with the other resident cat. The basement cat supposedly belonged to Sheila's son and was named "Sah" for reasons that were never clear to me. But when I began to ask questions about when he was going back to her son, I learned that the cat had resided in Sheila's basement for the past eight years. It was obvious that the cat was indeed going to be part of our household for the foreseeable future.

The other cat was a grouchy, but beautiful, longhaired Persian named Hedges (the cat prior was Benson). Hedges had been a long-time member of Sheila's household and could be described in many ways, friendly not being among them. He spent much of his day avoiding the presence of the dog who was quite convinced, according to Sheila, Hedges was a skunk worthy of a mad chase all over the house. How she knew what the dog thought about the cat was never clear to me, either.

Sheila's dog was named Honey, adopted as a puppy by Sheila and Allan. She was a Golden Retriever and was to be their "retirement dog." Honey's living arrangement was rather luxurious by dog standards, I thought. Our garage had a separate little storage room in it that had been converted to a home for Honey. She had a bed, food, water and a little doggie door that provided access out to a fenced-in area in the yard that was at least ten feet by ten feet with a little protected house and, believe it or not, a brick patio that had been built by Allan himself for Honey's enjoyment. The little garage room also had a space heater that Sheila would plug in for short periods of time on very cold winter nights. That dog lived better than do many children in the world.

I had two cats, Amos and Simon. Simon was ill with a thyroid condition that was expected to be fatal within the next several months. That sick cat was also prone to anxiety and nervousness. In my Pennsylvania house Simon was the one who would flee to the basement, leap up on a high wall and crawl on top of a heating duct every time my toddler-aged nephew and niece would come to visit. In Ohio he raced wildly to the basement and flew into the crawl space when unfamiliar people came around. Sometimes, he would not reappear for days.

Amos, my other cat, was more typical. Through the years with Amos, Sheila often said, "Amos is the best cat I ever knew." Given this unusual menagerie, we were quite concerned about how things would go when we set up a household in which these cats, the dog, and two people would reside together for the first time. Initially, we decided that the resident basement cat would continue to stay there. After all, if you haven't been out of the basement for eight years, why start now? We also decided that the dog would stay out in the garage or in the yard for a period of time while the two new cats adjusted to their surroundings.

Everything went surprisingly well for several days until we decided that it was time for the dog to come into the house to meet everybody. Sheila was used to having Honey in with her during the day. She enjoyed her companionship and liked the perpetually interactive nature of a dog. I think it helped to assuage her loneliness after Allan's death and her own retirement.

One of the prized possessions that Sheila identified in our

process of sorting through our things was her baby grand piano. Sheila was a very talented musician and especially loved playing her piano. It sat in our living room with the lid opened, ready to project her beautiful music into the household.

On the day that we opened the garage door and Honey came into the house, Amos, who was usually unintimidated by most things and was dozing in a relaxed lull, was rudely awakened by the dog's clamor. He took off so fast in the classic terrorized cat run with his belly dragging along the floor that I lost track of him. Sheila lunged to grab hold of Honey who was prepared to treat Amos just like she was used to treating Hedges.

Meanwhile, Simon had found cover earlier because he was adjusting more slowly to his new surroundings and usually was already halfway under cover somewhere. Once order was restored and Honey was calmed, the search for Amos began. We looked everywhere—under every bed and behind every piece of furniture. We searched all the usual places that a person would look for a scared cat, but to no avail.

Then I walked into living room and saw Amos inside the lid of the baby grand piano. He was looking rather smug actually, as if quite satisfied with himself for having found a perch that he was quite sure a dog could not reach. But he was on the soundboard of the beautiful piano. It flashed through my mind that I should dig him out of here and never tell Sheila where I found him. But such deception didn't seem like a very mature way to begin what would hopefully be a very long arrangement. I decided to leave him there, find Sheila, and tell her where he was, hoping that she would not immediately wish that my cats and I would go back to where we came from.

I walked from the living room into the family room where Sheila was, and said, "Sheila, I found him but I don't think you're going to like where he is." She looked at me in surprise and said, "Where is he?"

I said, "Sheila, he is inside the piano." I knew from the look on her face that she did not understand what I meant so I said, "Follow me."

We went into the living room and, to her eternal credit, she said, "Can we get him out of there carefully?" And she laughed. There was no whining or crying or screaming or handwringing or anything when she discovered my cat inside her prized possession. I think I knew then that if we were ever to have problems, Sheila's being persnickety would not be the source.

Within days, it was time to take Simon to the veterinarian for the last time. Sheila insisted on accompanying me to do something I had never done before and which I knew would be excruciating. She was present, supportive, and shed tears just as I did when my beloved cat died. Her behavior set the standard for our future approach to providing support, comfort, and a loving presence to each other as we would navigate life's challenges.

After Simon died and we settled into our new existence, I began to learn the extent of Sheila's dedication to the animal kingdom. She was a committed bird feeder, something she had learned from her mother. Both of them were almost eager to traipse through inches of snow in howling winds to replenish the bird feeders in their back yards. Sheila taught me that the bird food supplies had to be maintained in metal garbage cans in the garage, that feeders needed to be cleaned regularly, and that there was a way to peacefully exist with curious and determined squirrels. I remember being amazed at her commitment to keeping those feeders full. And when I once commented on it she replied, "It is a responsibility that I take seriously. They are depending on me and I plan to be there for them."

I had never paid the slightest bit of attention to backyard birds other than to observe the beauty of an occasional male cardinal who was hard to ignore. But living with Sheila opened my eyes to the joy of observing visiting birds, their migratory patterns, their playfulness, and their beauty. She was quite good and well informed about identifying back yard birds, including the pesky ones that occasionally annoyed her. But she would usually catch herself in the midst of her annoyance and subsequently declare, "But they are all God's creatures and they're hungry too, so the least we can do is provide for them."

She especially loved the finches and bought a special sock feeder that hung in a tree right outside the kitchen window. She often stood there and commented on the beauty of those finches and how she loved to watch them come and go and change color with the seasons. It gave her great joy to observe her beloved finches out the kitchen window.

But I would soon learn that our household's involvement with animals was not to be limited to the backyard birds and household pets. One winter shortly after I had foot surgery, Sheila was taking me to an appointment. As we backed out of the driveway and headed for the street, I observed a little gray creature that was too far away to be identifiable. "Sheila," I said, "look over there. What is that?" She paused her driving activities long enough to take a look and could not identify the little creature either.

Neither of us gave it much thought until the next day, when we saw the little lump of fur in the backyard, and this time went out to investigate. We approached slowly (me limping on the surgically-repaired foot) and were soon able to determine that we had a lop-eared rabbit in our backyard.

He seemed to be relatively tame but did not allow us to get closer than several yards from him. Sheila immediately declared that this little rabbit was "a poor little thing and has to be hungry." While we were speculating how in the world a lop-eared rabbit had arrived in our yard, Sheila was plotting a care-giving strategy, unknown to me until later. I was being self-absorbed, interested mostly in getting back into the house to prop my foot up and resume drinking tea.

I thought I had persuaded her that the rabbit could fend for itself. I should have realized that I was not anticipating her next move correctly when she later expressed concern that a fox would eat the rabbit and "that will be the end of the poor little thing."

I actually forgot about the rabbit until one day when I returned home from work several weeks later and began the process of listening to Sheila about how her day had gone. We had quickly developed this pattern of listening to each other, usually over dinner, about the respective activities we had undertaken during the day. I was often glad to not be thinking about business problems anymore, so listening to Sheila about household events or her interests was a helpful way for me to maintain balance and some semblance of mental health.

On this particular day, Sheila reported that she had developed an approach to feeding our visiting rabbit. Sure enough, when she directed my attention to the back yard, there was our recycling bin on its side, in which Sheila placed things she had determined to be prime rabbit food. She had selected lettuce, carrots, and I'm not sure what else for his consumption. She was even more pleased to report that she had set these delectables out in the early morning and discovered later in the day that some had been eaten. She was so happy. She told me how concerned that she had been that this rabbit was out there suffering in this especially cold weather without anything to eat.

Sheila developed a new daily routine that included visits to the backyard to replenish food for our little guest and to test his limits for human proximity. This went on for more than a week. During our catch-up time at the end of each day, Sheila would report her progress to me, including her desire to see the rabbit up close so she could be sure he wasn't injured and in need of veterinary care. Dollar signs flashed into my head.

I remember that it was a Friday when I arrived home to Sheila's triumphant announcement, "I captured the rabbit! He's in a box in the basement. He's fine – not injured at all. I just took a towel out there with me today and walked up to him and picked him up. He didn't resist at all. Isn't that wonderful?" That was not my first thought.

While I could not help but share her enthusiasm at her accomplishment, the practical side of me began to have multiple thoughts very quickly: what were we going to do with a rabbit in a household that already had three cats and a dog, where were we going to keep this thing for the weekend, how does a person take care of a rabbit, how am I going to be kind-hearted to my closest friend who has just fallen for a rabbit when I think that keeping a rabbit is absolutely crazy? I tried to slow my thoughts, took time to make positive comments to Sheila about the wonders of having rescued an abandoned rabbit, and then said, "Where do you think he should spend the night?"

I thought that was a very sensible way to start the practical conversation. Her immediate response was, "I don't know, but aren't you glad he's in the house and not out there in the cold?" Not really, but I was trying to be.

She did declare that the basement residence had to be temporary because that was "Sah's home" and we had to be concerned that a cat and a rabbit might not mingle very well overnight. I was quite glad to hear this line of thinking because the prospect of losing sleep over nocturnal animal activities in my basement was none too appealing. Then, after much discussion about not intruding on the dog's territory in the garage and the reality of our inability to properly house a rabbit in the house with us, Sheila agreed that the rabbit would stay in the garage.

But then she decided that it would need exercise.

"Sheila, are you kidding? This rabbit has gone from being a "poor little thing" to being a resident in our garage who needs exercise?"

She was absolutely certain that staying in a box was inhumane. So she insisted that we move our cars out of the garage to make a suitable home for this rabbit. Remember, it was late January in Ohio, not prime time to have a car in the driveway when you have a perfectly fine garage, to my way of thinking.

But this was her project and I wanted to be supportive, so I reluctantly agreed to move my car out of the garage. "Should I go get the rabbit from the basement now so we can get him settled in the garage?" I should have anticipated the next move.

"No! There are too many things in that garage that might hurt him. We have to go out there and inspect it to make sure he will be safe." Right. Just what I envisioned doing on a Friday evening in January—inspecting my own garage to be sure it meets Sheila's code for safely harboring a wayward rabbit. I tried to say that I thought the rabbit would be just fine on his own, but I wasn't making that sale. We ventured out, rearranged some things, (Sheila was especially concerned about some of my garden implements with sharp edges), moved the cars out, and moved the rabbit in. Sheila provided food and water and I envisioned cleaning up rabbit poop, an issue of no consequence to my rescuer friend at all.

On Saturday morning, after we confirmed that everyone in the household had survived the night intact, I began a conversation about a longer term plan regarding our rabbit guest. Fortunately, Sheila did agree that we were not equipped to have a rabbit nor did we see a way for us to become rabbit owners. But she qualified her agreement by making sure I shared her opinion that we would keep the rabbit as long as necessary until a proper home for him could be found. I did agree with that, especially after all of her impressive rescue efforts on behalf of this poor creature.

We soon settled on a plan to contact the Humane Society to see if they would take a rabbit. Meanwhile, I was being grouchy about the need to limp around in the snow in the driveway to get into my freezing cold car in order to go anywhere. Sheila was completely unconcerned about the inconvenience to herself of having her car in the driveway instead of in the garage—because the rabbit was warm and safe. From my perspective, we had at least settled on a plan to be in a holding pattern with this rabbit until he could be delivered to the Humane Society on Monday.

I was wrong. When we returned home from church on Sunday, Sheila informed me that two different families with young children were coming to the house in the afternoon to visit the garage rabbit. "Sheila, are you kidding? You have invited friends to come and visit the rabbit? Won't visitors interrupt his exercise routine? What about our commitment to spend our Sunday afternoons in a quiet and restful way?"

Of course to Sheila, this was a circumstance which called for an exception to the restful Sunday afternoon routine. She had been telling the story of the rabbit's rescue and his subsequent residency in the garage and could not help herself. This was great fun and she found the opportunity to share with others irresistible.

We ended up with four adults, five children, and someone's grandmother at our house that afternoon to visit a rescued rabbit! Of course, Sheila being Sheila and ever full of hospitality, served cookies and beverages to all of the guests.

I was upstairs reading the newspaper. This was one of those times when we chose to do separate things in the same house. I wasn't angry or upset with her decision at all, nor was she with mine. We understood the differences in our personalities and gave each other room to act accordingly.

Thankfully, the Humane Society in Columbus did have a provision for sheltering and placing rabbits. Who knew? I had no idea that those good people provided such a service for animals beyond dogs and cats.

When I got home from the office on Monday, I parked my car in the snowy driveway grumbling all the while about that rabbit having overtaken my parking spot in the garage, Sheila reported her day's activities. She had been able to get the rabbit into a smaller box in her car and transport him. She said that they were very pleased to receive him and were amazed at his beauty and good health. They told her it would have been unlikely for him to survive the winter outside on his own, because of his vulnerability to predators or starvation. They thanked Sheila for rescuing him and bringing him to them for placement. My dear friend had accomplished something meaningful, at some inconvenience to herself. But she did not even notice the inconvenience because it was all in the interest of helping another being. And I was only beginning to understand the extent to which this attitude of hers would eventually impact my own.

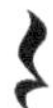

Over the next several years we experienced the death of Sah and Hedges and, ultimately—the best cat Sheila ever knew—the incomparable Amos. Eight years into our household arrangement, the only pet we had was the aging dog Honey. Sheila was very attached to Honey. Her typical routine involved reading the morning paper and drinking her coffee while seated in her favorite comfortable chair dressed in her night clothes. When she was ready to begin the active part of her day, Sheila would invite Honey in from her garage home and they would go upstairs for Honey to supervise Sheila's early day routine. Once emails were checked and the morning toilette completed, the two of them set off on their daily walk.

The entire neighborhood knew Sheila and Honey because both of them were so friendly. Honey's Golden Retriever personality and Sheila's interest in people were magnetic. They even became buddies with the grounds crew that maintained the large city park across the road from our house. Sheila learned all the men's names and they brought treats for Honey along in their maintenance trucks so they could interact with her when they met. Living with extroverts was providing a view into the world that was remarkable to this introvert.

In the winter of 2001, we hosted a small dinner party to celebrate the 60th birthday of a friend. One of the couples present had rescued a cat at their rural home. They described him as being a friendly cat that was determined to live inside of their house with them. The problem with that arrangement was the presence of their teenage daughter's cat, Chloe. This newly-arrived cat, named Tubbs because he was growing so large, was presenting a problem for that family. They decided to try to find a new home for him. Knowing that our household was catless, they asked us if we would take him. We agreed to think about it, partly because we missed having a cat and partly because we could be helpful to them.

After some brief discussion the next day, Sheila and I agreed that we would take the cat. Sally, the rescuer, invited us to come and visit the cat to be sure we were comfortable with him. We declined that offer and assured her that things would work out just fine. She had described his friendly personality and black and gray features enough for us to be comfortable. Because Sally felt responsible for taking the cat to the veterinarian for his initial shots and neutering operation, we agreed to pick him up at the vet's office when his various treatments were finished.

Everything was arranged for a Thursday of the following week. We bought cat food, a new litter box, and food bowls for the impending arrival. When I arrived home from work two days before the planned arrival of the new cat, I walked into our kitchen from the garage and saw a little black cat seated on the floor looking up at Sheila who was standing at the counter looking at me.

I immediately wondered how we could have confused the pick-up time for the new cat and looked at Sheila quizzically. It also flashed through my mind that this cat did not match the description Sally had given of a black, gray, and white cat.

Before I could say anything Sheila said, "Look, I found this poor little cat today. Isn't it cute? I was sweeping the garage and heard a small cry. It was across the street. I called to it and it just came running right to me. I had to bring it in the house. Look how hungry it is," she said, while dumping some of our newly purchased cat food into a bowl on the floor. That poor cat attacked that food in a way that I have never seen a cat do before. This cat had clearly been in a desperate situation.

Ever the practical one in the face of Sheila's soft heartedness, I asked her what she had in mind for this cat. "Well," she said, "I'm not sure. I don't know if you want to keep it. I suppose we could take it to the Humane Society but you would have to do that. I just couldn't possibly stand to do that. And I don't think I could stand to turn it back out into the cold."

She obviously knew how to appeal to my softer side. I quickly reviewed the advantages and disadvantages of another cat while trying to figure out how to not burst Sheila's bubble of enthusiasm over this. We had already planned to bring a cat into our house so we were equipped to have a feline pet. I laughed to myself at the folly of Sheila rescuing this animal and then announcing that she couldn't possibly take it to the Humane Society, so if we didn't want to keep it, I was on the hook to do the clean-up.

We briefly discussed the pros and cons of taking in another animal at this time. Not surprisingly, Sheila's argument was that there was not much difference between one cat and two cats. And after all, at one time our household had four cats so this would be no big deal. That logic was hard to argue with and it was obvious that Sheila was already attached to this little thing. So I suggested that if Sheila was willing to take the cat to the veterinarian as soon as possible to be sure that it would not spread any disease to the other cat we were expecting, we would keep it. Sheila did not hesitate one moment before agreeing to that plan.

The next day when I got home from the office, Sheila reported on her visit to the veterinarian earlier in the day. With the cat not even having a name, the veterinarian's office created a folder with the label "Stray" on it. Sheila said that when the doctor came into the examination room after having read that label, her eyes got very wide and after one glance at the cat, she said; "Wow a pure-bred Persian cat is not usually a stray. This cat is quite valuable."

The veterinarian's judgment after examining the cat, was that she had been out on her own for many weeks. Sheila, of course, lamented at how anyone could possibly abandon any cat, not to mention someone as lovely as this. We later made some efforts to find the owner, to no avail.

From the visit to the vet, Sheila reported the cat to be not only quite feisty, but also to have ear mites, fleas, an eye infection, nutritional deficiencies, and a suspected respiratory infection. This of course required much treatment and extensive plans for follow-up visits. It was also determined that the cat was a female. For my money, it was also the most expensive stray cat in history.

We had been debating the name of the male cat whose arrival we had planned for the following day. Half-joking I said that I didn't think we should retain the name Tubbs because I thought it would be harmful to the cat's self-esteem. Sheila readily agreed with that. Thus, we decided to honor the cat's heritage and his prior family's name yet find a way to give him a name that would be pleasing for us. We finally decided on Ernest. Officially, his name was Earnest Tubbs but we would call him "Ernie."

Once that was decided, Sheila quickly labeled the new little feline girl "Blanche," fittingly inspired by the character from A Streetcar Named Desire who, Sheila reminded me, relied on the kindness of strangers.

Honey was more than happy to welcome these two new arrivals. Ernie was completely unintimidated by the dog and was able to interact with her in a way that was appropriate for any interaction between an eighty-five pound dog and a ten pound cat. Blanche, on the other hand, was deemed by Honey to be chase-able. This resulted in a series of mad dashes around the house reminiscent of Honey's interactions with Hedges. Blanche soon learned that when she heard that dog approaching from the garage, it was in her best interest to find a remote hiding place and stay there until the dog left. All in all, we settled into a new existence that was quite satisfactory for everyone—until the summer of 2003.

I was at the beach in New Jersey with my family for a week. I called Sheila early in the week just to check in and say hello. She reported that Honey was having digestive problems and she was taking her to the veterinarian. Sheila knew that Honey was fading, as the poor dog had developed arthritis and was generally in a declining condition that could be expected for a large dog of fourteen. Sheila dreaded Honey's passing. I know there were many nostalgic thoughts about the dog because Sheila and Allan had selected her as a puppy, adapted their home to meet her needs, trained and enjoyed her in her early years. And Sheila often told me how helpful it was to have Honey around after Allan died, except when the dog searched and searched for Allan and missed him. This behavior compounded Sheila's grief but on the whole, she treasured the dog's company.

Thus, I was distressed to learn, later in the week when I called, that Honey's condition did not improve over several days after the visit to the veterinarian. Ultimately, Sheila made the decision to have the dog put down. The veterinarian came to our house and in our front hallway, with Sheila by her side, Honey died. Sheila chose to have her cremated and her ashes returned to us.

I felt terrible being so far away and leaving Sheila to deal with this alone. But this experience was a good example of her strength. She was decisive and very capable of managing a challenging situation. In this case, she made the necessary decisions and followed through on her plan of action.

When I got home, she filled me in on all the details of what had happened and I shared her sorrow at the loss of her much loved dog. She told me that her plan was to scatter Honey's ashes in the park across the street where they had spent so many days enjoying their walks. She wasn't ready to do that right away, but when she was, I asked if she wanted me to come along. She did. I was honored. We took a nice walk on a perfect late summer day, reminiscing about Honey's good days in the park. Sheila scattered the ashes, shed a few quiet tears, and we walked home together.

Sheila did not miss having a dog until the temperatures cooled and conditions were perfect for morning walks. After Honey died, we were busy hosting house guests, taking a vacation, and handling various early fall church activities. But when all of that died down, Sheila began taking walks alone and she did not like it one bit. She really missed the companionship of a dog at the end of a leash as she strolled through the neighborhood, across the road, and into the park each day.

She casually mentioned one evening that maybe it would be nice to have another dog. But then she thought for a moment and said she was not sure she really wanted to do all of the work required to have one. I don't remember saying much of anything because I am a cat person, not a dog person. I was learning quite a bit about the realities of living with a dog but did not feel really compelled to have another one in the house.

As Sheila provided her updates to me at the end of each day during this time, she often told me about taking a walk and how "dreadful" it was without the dog. This went on for several weeks until I finally suggested that we look into getting another dog. Again, Sheila mentioned her hesitation to take on the work required with having a dog. Privately, I was wondering if I was losing my mind by suggesting that we bring a new dog into the household. However, Sheila seemed to miss the presence of a dog and I thought she should have one if it meant a lot to her. This is what I told her.

After some additional back and forth conversations about the merits of getting another dog, we noticed an invitation in the newspaper to a special open house at the local Humane Society. They were undertaking an extra effort to have their overcrowded conditions relieved by encouraging adoption of some of their resident pets. I suggested to Sheila that we visit the Humane Society "just to look around." She continued to be hesitant about bringing anther dog into our house but agreed that there was nothing to lose by visiting the Humane Society.

So, on a Friday night that fall, we piled into Sheila's car and took off. During the ride, Sheila described the kind of dog she preferred. She wanted an animal that was not small and "yippy" nor too large for her to handle. She wanted a dog with a "silky" coat and a friendly demeanor. The new dog also had to be a female because the male leg-lifting process for urine elimination was offensive to my friend for some reason. None of this mattered to me whatsoever. I kept telling her that if she wanted to have a dog, we should get a dog.

We arrived at the Humane Society, parked the car, and walked across the parking lot into a teeming mass of people with dogs on leashes. The weather was perfect, the volunteer dog walkers enthusiastic, and the dogs apparently enjoying themselves. None of the volunteers were pushy in any way. They simply walked the dogs around in the large open area and waited for people to approach. Almost immediately, Sheila noticed a black dog being walked by a woman some distance away. She commented that the dog was a nice size and seemed to be friendly. We ventured closer to them and Sheila asked about the dog's name. "It's 'Hildey,'" the woman replied. Sheila immediately commented that she liked the name and began to interact with the dog.

Sheila then disengaged from talking to Hildey and the handler with a comment about our intent to just look around. We strolled through the general area observing different dogs at play with both their handlers and other visitors enjoying the whole affair. As we walked, I asked Sheila if she saw a dog here that she would like to adopt. Her eyes looked past me into the distance where Hildey was enjoying herself with her handler. "I would take that one if I were going to take one," she said. "She seems just right and I would feel terrible thinking about her spending the rest of her life at the Humane Society. But we said we were just going to look around so let's just go home." I knew that she was saying this because she was aware of my lukewarm feelings about having a dog around. Yet I truly felt that she should have another dog even if I was lukewarm about it.

"Sheila," I said "I think we should take Hildey home with us if she is the dog you would like. I know you are worried about handling the work as you get older, but I will help you. If you are willing to train the dog and integrate her into our household, let's do this."

After several additional moments of deliberation, Sheila finally said, "Well, I guess Ernie would like it if he had another dog to play with." I cracked up. This was classic Sheila, finding a way to be sure that her actions would help somebody else. In this case, she knew it wouldn't be me, but was happy to nominate poor Ernie. We agreed to take Hildey home.

I asked myself how could two people who were usually quite precise in making plans have set out on this expedition without thinking about the possibility of actually returning with a dog? After Honey died, Sheila had gotten rid of her food, bed, leash, and feeding bowls. Here we were about to take a dog to our house with no means to really properly care for her. We knew we had paperwork to do to finalize the adoption and as it was getting late, we realized that a stop on the way home for dog supplies would be essential to the successful survival of everyone on Hildey's first night with us.

With paperwork completed, and Hildey becoming more excited by the moment (no doubt taking her cues from Sheila), we headed across the parking lot toward the car with the volunteer dog walker. Sheila decided that she would sit in the back seat with the dog to "begin the bonding process." Obviously, my role was to drive. As we clamored into the car, I reminded Sheila that we needed dog supplies. Yes, she knew of a Walmart close by that would still be open.

It flashed through my mind that this was completely crazy. I had not envisioned myself racing down the highway to Walmart on a Friday night with my closest friend and an excitable dog positioned as backseat drivers. I prompted Sheila to make a list of essential supplies so we could be efficient once we arrived at the store, but she was preoccupied by her bonding activities in the back seat and was rather absently telling me some things we would need.

When we arrived at Walmart, things became more serious. "Okay Sheila," I said, "why don't I stay with the dog while you go get the supplies we need?"

"Oh no," she said. She wanted to stay with the dog. It was important to establish the "leader of the pack" bond that she had apparently been working on already in the back seat. While it seemed highly unlikely to me that disruption of these activities for a few short moments would in any way be a problem for the long term relationship with the dog, Sheila was quite sure that she needed to stay with Hildey and I had to go into the store.

"Terrific. Tell me what we need."

We made a list, with Sheila offering very specific instructions on certain things. I ventured off thinking that I wanted to get these supplies, get us safely home, get those two out of the back seat of the car, and survive the night, hopefully without a dog barking hysterically the entire time.

I bought toys, having lost the argument that toys were not essential for surviving the night (The dog needed the presence of her new toys in order to relax, I was told), a bed, food, food bowls, and a leash. By now, I was the one not relaxed. Nevertheless, we made it and Sheila just loved her new dog. They took walks, developed a similar daily routine to the previous one with Honey, and involved Ernie in their usual canine-feline interactions.

Blanche was completely put off by dogs thanks to Honey's chasing tendencies, so she found safe hiding places and we all adjusted. Sheila took Hildey to obedience school and practiced with her daily. Hildey adapted quite well to Honey's former domain in the garage and the yard. We had few problems. Until I had to take over dog duties.

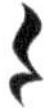

In the spring of the following year, Sheila hurt her foot. The orthopedic doctor prescribed rest and a walking boot that she was supposed to wear for several weeks. When I arrived home to learn this news, Sheila included a casual comment about how it was too bad that Hildey hadn't had a walk that day. She really was not being manipulative, but for me, it was a clue to offer to walk the dog that evening. She accepted my offer, provided a few tips on Hildey's tendencies, and off we went after I finished the dinner dishes.

Our route took us through the neighborhood, across the road, and into the park. Passing through the neighborhood, my thoughts were mostly random until I passed one home where an occasionally unpleasant lady lived. Mindy G. seemed to have little to do other than mind everyone else's business. Her demeanor was often sour and her comments about people in the neighborhood were rarely positive. She was touchy and fussy and I had to think she was mostly unhappy. I was hoping she wasn't outside because interactions with her were just usually long and uncomfortable. We passed by her house uneventfully.

When Hildey and I returned from our walk, the dog bounded into the house ahead of me and ran to greet Sheila. I followed closely behind. "How did it go?" Sheila asked.

"It was great. Hildey pooped in Mindy G's yard!" I announced triumphantly.

Sheila instantly struggled to her feet with a look of horror on her face. "Did you pick it up?" she asked.

"What?" I said, "Did I pick it up? Why would I have done that?"

"Oh." Sheila said, "I should have sent you with a plastic bag so you could pick it up if she pooped. We have to go get it."

"Sheila, are you serious? We have to go get the dog poop?"

By this time she was grabbing her car keys and limping toward the door to the garage. I was thinking that this was the craziest thing I could imagine—driving down the street and stopping the car to pick up dog poop from grouchy Mindy's yard.

"We are seriously going to go pick up dog poop from Mindy G.'s yard?"

"Yes!" Sheila said emphatically "We have to go get it. You cannot leave dog poop in someone else's yard. I should have told you that. We have to go right now before she finds it!"

As I was trying to suggest something terribly unkind about the appropriateness of the dog's deposit in Mindy's yard, Sheila was moving past me as fast as she could go toward the garage door with her keys, grabbing a plastic grocery bag from the sleeve that hung in our pantry. It was obvious that this was not a topic for further discussion.

I realized that if I did not go along, my friend who was supposed to be resting her foot would be traipsing around in Mindy's yard in search of dog poop. If she was going to defy doctor's orders, I did not think this circumstance should be the one she should be explaining to the doctor.

"Do you know exactly where it is?" Sheila asked as she stepped into the garage with me trailing close behind.

Not having realized that I should have committed the exact spot to memory, I said, "I think I know the general area."

By the time I got into the garage, Sheila had the door open, the car started, and had shifted into reverse as I jumped into the passenger seat. She was not angry, just concerned that a breach of dog etiquette was in the works because she had not properly schooled me in dog walking procedures. As we raced down the street to Mindy's house, Sheila quickly coached me on the finer points of picking up dog poop with a grocery bag wrapped around one's hand.

Fortunately, it was getting dark with less chance of my being seen and I was able to locate the offensive poop quickly. Mindy never knew we were there as far as we could tell—and much to Sheila's relief.

As we arrived back at our house with the grocery bag of goods, I said; "Now what do we do with it?" Obviously, this entire process was completely unknown to me.

"Put it in the garbage can," Sheila coached.

Never again did I take the dog for a walk without a question ringing in my ears, "Do you have a grocery bag with you?" And never again will I forget the courtesy of respecting other persons' property, even if they are grouchy.

Personalities

One component of the leadership training I received at the large insurance company where I worked was an introduction to the Myers-Briggs Personality Indicator. My profile, in Myers-Briggs was INTJ. The company believed it was important for people in leadership roles to know their own tendencies and to recognize the value of different tendencies in coworkers. When I told Sheila about this and described how useful I thought it was to have these understandings, she was immediately interested in learning her own personality type. Not surprising, Sheila turned out to be an ESFP, the exact opposite of me.

We knew very well that we were quite different before our exposure to the personality assessment tool. But it provided useful language for us to use at home when our differences might have resulted in tension.

I occasionally pointed out to Sheila that my introverted self needed some quiet time for a while before we moved on to whenever our plans were just as she reminded me of her need for interaction and socializing with others. I soon discovered that living with someone so different from me could be entertaining.

One evening during our typical dinner conversation, Sheila mentioned that she had received a very interesting telephone call that day. "It was a wrong number," she said.

I had a very hard time imagining how a wrong number telephone call could possibly be interesting, so I waited for additional information.

"It was a ninety-year-old woman who thought she was calling her daughter. She was a little bit confused and I felt sorry for her, so I talked to her for a while." She then proceeded to tell me that this woman had grown up in southern Ohio, not far from where Sheila herself lived as a child, that the woman was a retired teacher, and was living in the Columbus area. Sheila also shared some details about the woman's medical history, educational career, and extended family.

I finally asked, "Sheila, how long did this conversation go on?"

"Oh," she said "I think it was only about forty minutes."

"Sheila, you're kidding! You spent forty minutes on the phone today with a wrong number?" thinking that such a call would consume no more than thirty seconds of my time, if I'd have answered the phone at all.

"Well," she replied, "the woman was very interesting and needed someone to talk to and I had some time. She was embarrassed that she dialed the wrong number and I think she felt better by the end of the conversation."

I'm sure she did. And Sheila is the only person I know who could possibly spend forty minutes talking to a wrong number caller.

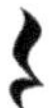

Visits by repair people were also occasions that reminded me of the differences in our personality types. Typically, Sheila made the appointments and opened our door to the plumber, furnace maintenance guy, painter, Orkin inspector, or anyone else who needed access to our home to provide services. Despite my offers to arrange my schedule to be at home for this purpose, Sheila insisted that it made more sense for her to handle these things since she was retired and had more flexibility in her schedule. And so it was.

A typical conversation at the end of a day when someone who provided service had visited went like this,

> "Sheila, what did the (plumber furnace guy, painter, ….) say about the (pipes, furnace, paint job, bugs….)?"
>
> "Everything is fine," she would say, "but the whole thing took so much longer than I thought it would. I had other things to do today and didn't get to as many as I would have liked to."
>
> "So, Sheila, is there a problem with the (pipes, furnace…) that made everything take longer?"
>
> "No, but Joe (or Frank or Harry or whoever) was here. I think he's been here before. He's thinking about retiring and his wife (or mother or daughter or someone) has been sick and he's very worried. He's (been working a lot of overtime, hurt his leg, sick himself….). He's from (insert any city) and we got to talking about (insert tourist attraction, someone they both knew, recent news about the area)."

Initially, I had a hard time understanding how such information could possibly be elicited from a repair person. As time went on and I became more attuned to my extrovert friend, her interest in people and need to interact with them no matter the circumstance, I was no longer surprised by these conversations.

Sometimes when Sheila would complain about the time these visits took, I would say something like, "Sheila, let's review your interaction with this person. You're complaining about the time it took but I'll bet you asked the questions, didn't you? Surely, the furnace guy did not walk into the house and start telling you about his retirement plans or his sick mother. You asked, right?"

She would grudgingly admit that she started these conversations about the personal lives of the repair people.

I would say, "If you want the visit to involve only business, don't ask the personal questions. I don't have the faintest idea whether the Orkin guy is planning a vacation to Mali or not."

I didn't really expect that anything would change and, over time, I came to understand that Sheila's interactions with repair people were as much a part of who she was as was my being brief and businesslike with them.

I used to detect a note of disappointment when the men came to the house and discovered me there rather than her. I don't think I was ever rude or curt with them, but their disappointment eventually caused me to work at overcoming my own tendencies to "get down to work" and spend a bit more time showing interest in people.

One of the agreements Sheila and I made from the very beginning was to share our house with friends and family. It was a large two-story rectangle on two-thirds of an acre, at the end of a dead-end street. The first floor had living room and dining room in the front, with kitchen, eating area, and family room in the back. Beside the kitchen, on the way to the garage was a half bath and laundry room. The second floor had two full baths and five bedrooms.

Sheila and Allan had built the house in the mid-1960's when Allan had taken a new job as band director at the local high school. They moved from a smaller area and decided to build the home that would accommodate their three children and visiting grandparents who had all retired in Florida. So when visitors from Florida came for nice long visits in the summer, there was a bedroom for everyone.

We arranged its second-floor use with three bedrooms, an office, and what we called the "sitting room" upstairs where one of us could retreat if the other was doing something downstairs from which we wanted to be removed. That room also contained a sofa-bed that came in handy when we had many house guests.

Knowing Sheila's generous spirit before I ever moved in, I did make her promise that she would check with me before taking in any wayward folks who needed a place to be for the long haul. That would have pushed me far out of my comfort zone and disrupted my need to have my house be a place for some solitude. Sheila readily agreed, pledging quite seriously that she was unlikely to adopt either strangers or hard-luck distant relatives at this stage of her life. But I knew she had done so in the past.

Over the years, we kept our commitment to share what we had. We hosted many parties (Olympics, hymn sings, holidays, birthdays, game nights, OSU vs PSU football games) and housed many visitors, mostly my relatives and friends from Pennsylvania. Occasionally, Sheila's brother would visit from Alabama. And we once had a slumber party of local friends followed a year or two later by the same with four of her childhood friends. In both cases, otherwise mature sensible women acted like we were in college again, except that recovery took longer.

We developed a rather predictable routine for planning and executing these get-togethers. Sheila was an excellent cook and enjoyed having guests. She felt like it was a way of showing love and she was good at it. Being more practical and not terribly interested in culinary pursuits, I usually handled logistics (chairs, tables, errands, coats) with the understanding that my most serious job, especially during dinner parties, was to keep guests out of Sheila's kitchen.

She was not a multitasker and took her food preparations quite seriously. She pleaded with me to keep people away from the kitchen while she did last-minute preparations. The rule always was that we did everything. ("It's not a treat for people to go out to a dinner party if they have to take something. This is our party, we'll do it.') Her preparations required her full attention and exquisite timing. She was sure that people talking to her would only result in calamity, so my little introverted self had to become the conversationalist extraordinaire until the food preparations were complete and people were invited to the table.

Sheila kept detailed notes on her menus and maintained those notes so that, if a group returned for another visit, she could refer to her book to be sure she did not serve the same thing again. Apparently, that would be unthinkable. I tried to argue that nobody would notice or care; they would just be glad to be there eating her food. But this was a point of pride with Sheila and she really worked at it and enjoyed it.

She spent hours arranging the table settings to be just perfect for whatever occasion. "Presentation is everything," was her mantra and she did things up right. She acknowledged a weakness for purchasing table coverings and used her stash with a keen eye.

Fresh seasonal flowers from my flower gardens in our yard were often included.

People loved to come to our house and we worked at making them feel very special and valued during and after their visits. My Ohio friends and I still sometimes recall with great fondness Sheila's refrain that "presentation is everything," while also recognizing the unmitigated joy that comes from the presence of friends and family, no matter the presentation.

On the occasion of my approaching fiftieth birthday, Sheila told me that she "really, really" wanted to have a surprise birthday party for me, but she was pretty sure I would not like that. She was right. She instead proposed an arrangement where I knew there would be a party, but specifics would be a secret.

I could see that she relished the possibilities so I agreed to cooperate and promised to impose no limits on her plans other than gifts. I insisted that I absolutely would not cooperate with stupid old-age gag gifts, nor did I want our friends to buy me gifts. I already had plenty of stuff, bought myself whatever I needed or wanted, and did not want to spend the day after a party figuring out what to do with the gift loot. Sheila agreed to these terms. I held my breath. I could tell that she was enjoying her party preparations immensely. Some of that was because she could torment me about what I didn't know and some if it was because she just loved planning parties.

On the day of the event, she told me to dress casually and be ready to get in the car at 5:00. I should have known that she had not planned a small dinner party at our house. I had to remember that this was an extrovert in action.

At the appointed hour, we left our house, headed out of the neighborhood and turned up the road on which our church was located. As Sheila drove into the church driveway, I suddenly noticed that, on the church lawn were at least thirty cardboard Holstein cow figures somehow attached thereto, scatted about in random fashion looking just like an actual miniature grazing herd.

"Sheila, there is a herd of cows on the church lawn. Surely, you didn't…."

Before she could reply, I next noticed that the parking lot contained many cars. Oh, my. She had invited a small army to this party.

"Yes, the party has a heifer theme and you'll understand why later," she declared with clear delight. I was starting to wonder if I had lost my mind when I agreed to cooperate with this madness.

The heifer theme was not surprising coming from her. Sheila had been a music teacher at the elementary school level for nearly twenty five years. A teaching device that she created early in her career was to introduce a character named "Mrs. Cow." Sheila had grown up on a dairy farm and loved the cows and was still drawn to them. I noticed it when we drove through rural areas and she would comment on the beauty of the cows in the field. She enjoyed pictures of cows and artwork that contained cows. I'm not sure of the appeal. She could not describe it exactly either. "I just like them. Look at their faces."

I'm not sure exactly how Mrs. Cow contributed to children learning music, but apparently she did. And she took on a life of her own. She became quite famous in the school building. Sheila had a small stuffed cow, named Mrs. Cow, who resided on the piano in her school room. She had personalized license plates on her car that read "MRSCOW." (I remember seeing that plate in the church parking lot when I first attended the church and wondered who "Mr. Scow" was.)

Sheila had a Christmas tree full of cow ornaments that children had given her over the years. She had knick-knacks galore from her adult friends who all knew about her affinity for cows. She even kissed a live cow that a farmer brought to the school parking lot when the school's children achieved a reading goal that, if accomplished, called for Mrs. Cow to kiss a cow as a reward for the children's achievement. Apparently the event was well staged and the Columbus newspapers published pictures of Sheila kissing the cow.

As we walked into the church fellowship hall, it was full of friends mingling and enjoying hors d'oeuvres and punch. Thank goodness Sheila did not have them hiding behind chairs poised to yell "surprise" when I showed up. I think she knew that would be too much.

As we concluded a very agreeable meal, Sheila took a microphone and called the group to attention. ("Uh, oh – entertainment," I thought.) I wasn't too uncomfortable at such a prospect because I trusted Sheila—and she delivered. After some silly jokes and funny stories poking fun at me by the MC she had turned the program over to, there was a clamor from a back room in the hall. Out came Sheila dressed head to toe in a cow costume, complete with synthetic udder.

The crowd applauded loudly as the MC announced a visit from

Mrs. Cow. Sheila went to the piano. She proceeded to belt out several songs whose words she had modified for the occasion to poke fun at me, singing in her special Mrs. Cow voice to the delight of the group.

Of course, I had heard about Mrs. Cow and had asked Sheila to do her entertainment bit for me, but she had always declined, stating that Mrs. Cow retired when she retired from teaching. I was now touched that she not only did all the work to arrange the party (where did she get those cardboard cows!), but she took time to buy a cow costume and work up a routine in my honor. This friend was a real keeper and I sometimes wondered if I deserved her.

There was more. When we arrived, I had not noticed a little table near the door on which there was a small basket. As the festivities wound down, Sheila took the microphone, thanked everyone for coming (this was after I said a few words of appreciation), and announced to me that, in lieu of gifts, our friends had been invited to make contributions in honor of my birthday to Heifer International, a charity I had long supported, but which had been new to Sheila.

She loved it when I had told her about Heifer International several years prior. With her affinity for cows, and the outstanding work of the Heifer organization to provide animals and training to people in developing countries so their lives could be changed, Sheila had joined me in becoming an enthusiastic supporter of the charity.

When we got home and Sheila counted the contributions, we saw that our friends had given gifts in excess of $500. I immediately decided to match that and we were quite proud to send a donation to Heifer International that allowed for the purchase of two heifers—and all because I had agreed to cooperate with my party-planning friend.

Our personality types were not our only differences. Sheila had been raised in a family of musicians and artists. I was raised in a family of athletes and sports fans. Sheila's mother attended Columbus symphony concerts as a season ticket holder until shortly before her death at age ninety-one. We followed local, state, and national sports teams.

After Allan's death, Sheila, her daughter, and son-in-law attended the concerts with her mother. The first time this foursome was scheduled to attend one of the concerts, Sheila announced her planned departure time that was more than an hour before the start time. For a twenty-minute drive, parking close by, and reserved seats, I didn't get it. "Sheila, why are you leaving so early?"

She looked at me rather incredulously, "Because you have to allow for toddle time."

"Toddle time?"

"Yes my mother is approaching ninety years of age. She needs time to toddle into my car, then into the concert hall and to our seats, with a bathroom stop beforehand. She always stops at the lounge, mostly to be sure her hair looks good in case she meets the maestro in the elevator again. That happened one time a few years ago and she was so thrilled. We'll be lucky if this is enough time."

Sheila always came home from those symphony concerts highly stimulated. Sometimes her eyes would fill with tears when she told me about a particularly beautiful section of music from some composer's symphonic work. She usually added the historical background of the piece which added to her ability to appreciate the music. She rarely complained about any music, only occasionally saying something like, "Schumann isn't my favorite but the orchestra did a very nice job, especially the strings. And my mother liked it." This would qualify as a highly satisfying evening for my friend.

I soon learned that Sheila's classical music preferences leaned toward the more romantic Russian composers, especially Rachmaninov because she loved those piano concertos. She also favored Mozart and Chopin.

Sheila was a naturally gifted pianist. She played by ear, which meant that having music in front of her was distracting and disruptive. It was enlightening to learn about this gift of hers. If she knew a tune or heard one several times, she could immediately play it on the piano with full chords, interesting adaptations of her own, and no hesitation.

She also had a certain look on her face when she was at the piano. It was not exactly concentration and it certainly wasn't any kind of anxiety or strain, as would have been the case for me. I think it was absorption. She was taken in by the music and what her mind enabled her fingers to do. I once asked her what she was thinking when she sat down to play the piano like that. It seemed to me that she had to be thinking about what chords to play or how the song went or something and I suggested that in my question to her.

"No," she said. "You're not the first person to ask me that. Allan couldn't understand it either. The best way I can think to describe it is that it's like reading. Do you think about how to read while you're reading? I don't think about the music when I'm playing, I just know how to play."

Okay, I thought. Sometimes, it's best to just accept the wonder of God's gift to someone because analysis minimizes the ability to just appreciate it.

Sheila's musical mindset created the context for her experiences of the world around her. She was extremely attuned to birdsongs, animal sounds, and disruptive sounds like lawn mowers, power tools, or airplanes. This sometimes manifested itself in ways that provided great entertainment both for me and for our friends who enjoyed listening to my tales of Sheila's latest "wacko musician" (my favorite reference for her) experiences.

One evening when we were sitting in our family room reading and watching television, Honey began to bark in the garage. This was not particularly unusual, as she sometimes did that to get attention in the hope that she would be re-admitted to the household for the evening. Usually when her barking efforts were unsuccessful, she quieted down after a short while. On this occasion, however, Honey persisted. Sheila, who always seemed to know what animals were thinking, declared, "She wants to come in because I was gone all day today and she missed me."

I didn't say anything since I most likely would have said something less than constructive. I did not believe that Sheila could read the mind of a dog. So I kept quiet, Honey kept barking, and her owner kept fretting about the dog's persistence. I could see that Sheila was getting more and more agitated by Honey's behavior and I suggested that she just bring the dog into the house for a while.

"No, then she'll think that she can come in every evening (I found this very hard to believe), and we don't want to start that. The usual routine is best. Dogs like routine."

Right, I thought, as I glanced at Ernie lounging nearby. He seemed to have a slightly smug expression on his face that I attributed to his assessing this situation and feeling privileged to be in the house while the dog was relegated to the garage to beg for attention. I'll take a smug cat any day.

The barking persisted and Sheila announced her intention to ignore the dog until she stopped barking. "She'll quit soon," she said more to convince herself than me, I think. I was not saying anything. Managing Honey was her job. Neither one of us said anything while the dog continued to bark. I knew Sheila was very bothered by both the noise and her adored dog's discontentment. But the plan was to wait her out, so I went back to reading the newspaper while my anxious friend pretended to be watching television. I suspected that Sheila wanted to bring the dog in but did not want to reverse her plan partly because she knew I would tease her about her soft heart for her dog.

I peeked over the paper once while Honey was being especially loud. Sheila caught my eye and announced, "I can't stand this. If she's going to bark for such a long time, the least she could do is change key!" I cracked up and Sheila had to laugh in spite of her frustration. But she was seriously bothered by the repetitive tone of the noise.

"Sheila, I'll go right out there and talk to Honey about barking in another key for a while—and I'll take her a treat. She's not expecting me, so maybe just a little attention from someone will help. And you can get relief from whatever key she's been in." I thereby found myself kneeling on the floor of my own garage feeding a biscuit to a dog whose inability to bark in several keys was annoying her owner.

Honey did calm down after a little bit of attention. As a matter of pride and conscience, I refused to have the conversation with her about changing key. Some things were just not understandable for Honey and me, but we were together on this one. Honey and I had not spent much time together, but we did a mini bonding thing that night. I believe I detected a look of distain from Ernie when I came back into the house.

Sheila and I were driving north on I-75 in Michigan on our way to a visit to Mackinac Island one summer, enjoying the kind of casual conversation and comfortable silences that happen easily between close friends. We enjoyed road trips and this one was especially welcome after some hectic times for both of us. We were looking forward to getting away for our first visit to the island.

As we drove along, and the conversation paused for a moment, Sheila said, "Bee," followed by silence. I waited for more words and then glanced sideways at her from the driver's seat when none were forthcoming. She had clearly said what she had to say but I was lost. For a moment, I thought I had allowed my mind to wander off thereby losing the flow of conversation. But that was unlikely since I was driving and had to keep my mind engaged on matters at hand. I also momentarily wondered if there was a bumble bee in the car that she was trying to make me notice, but it seemed that would have caused her to be more excited than her casual demeanor was. Clearly, the only thing to do was ask for clarification.

"What did you say, Sheila?" "Bee," she replied, with a continued look of some concentration on her face.

Still confused, I said, "Sheila, I think I missed something. What are you talking about?"

"I think it's a Bee."

"What is a bee?" Now I was getting frustrated trying to follow her, especially because she was not ordinarily a difficult conversationalist at all.

"That sound. I think it's a B, maybe B-flat."

"What sound?" The radio was not on and I was not hearing any music from anywhere.

"The sound the tires are making. I hope we get out of this cattle chute thing soon. It's getting annoying. Margie (a friend and musician at church) has perfect pitch. She would know for sure what note that is."

We were driving through a construction zone in which concrete barriers created temporary driving lanes. The lane we were in required us to drive on the rumble-strip type things that usually warn drivers that they were drifting off the side of the road. They were indeed causing a whine as we drove and Sheila was hearing it as a musical note! I was hardly noticing it at all, but my dear musician was in her world of sounds, a place I think most of us have never even visited.

Things could get very interesting when her world of sounds and the arts intersected with my world of athletics. Sheila was naturally curious and always willing to learn new things; when I invited her to share my life as a sports fan, she sometimes came along. Her observations were always as entertaining for me as were the actions in the competition. She needed no prompting to appreciate things like gymnastics ("Look at that form. Isn't the human body beautiful?") or figure skating ("that score [music!] is perfect for those movements"). But football and basketball were another matter—unless the slow motion of an athlete in full extension was shown, which would elicit the observation, "The human body is beautiful; that extension is just like ballet."

During the years when her granddaughter was in the local high school marching band, Sheila was very committed to attending the home games. The first time I was available to go along, I noticed that kick-off time was approaching and Sheila was being very casual about leaving the house. It was a very short distance to the high school, but it seemed to me that she was cutting it very close. That was unusual. Sheila did not like to be late for anything. I finally said something and she replied, "Oh, we don't have to rush. The home team's band doesn't play until halftime. We have plenty of time."

This prelude to our trip to the game should have alerted me to what would happen after the halftime band performance was finished. I had become interested in the game, which was very close with a rival school. But when the band exited the field, Sheila stood up and said, "OK, let's go. Intermission is over," which I took to mean a visit to the refreshment stand. But, no, she was ready to go home, having developed absolutely no interest in the football game despite having sat through much of the first half of a very good game. I soon learned that this was the routine of many "band followers" at a football game. It had never before occurred to me that someone would be interested in only the band.

And I don't know how many sporting events we watched or attended together where I had to remind her that, while musicians have "intermission," athletes refer to breaks as "halftime."

We also had to work on "rehearsal" and "practice." Frequently, I had to remind her that the Buckeye football players (she did have some interest in watching Buckeye football games, much to the considerable consternation of the Penn State Nittany Lion fan she lived with) did not think they were going to rehearsal every day.

One year for my birthday Sheila insisted that I provide suggestions on a gift she could provide. I resisted on the grounds that I didn't want or need anything more than I already had, but she persisted. I mentioned doing several things that I knew she would enjoy, but she rejected those options as "not being for your interests." Finally I suggested that we get tickets to see the Columbus professional ice hockey team play. I knew she couldn't argue with that one! And I really did want to go to a game.

Sheila jumped at the idea and, of course, found the possibility of a new adventure and planning an event to be quite stimulating. The team and the arena were relatively new to the city, so this was a unique experience all around.

At the game, I offered to explain some of the rules of ice hockey, but Sheila declined. "I'll just see what I can pick up as it goes along. Where are our boys trying to score a goal so I know where to look especially?"

I pointed out the net to our left and we settled in to watch the game. I could tell that Sheila was enjoying herself. She liked the energy in the building and the stimulating environment of a major league athletic event. Early in the game, when two players began an on-ice tussle, she laughed. This seemed like a very unusual response from someone who consistently distained violence and confrontation. I asked, "Sheila, why are you laughing at these guys fighting?"

"Listen to the music!" she replied and looked at me like I was missing a highlight of the evening. "It's 'Why Can't We Be Friends'! Isn't that wonderful? What a sense of humor! I didn't know there would be organ music here. Where is the organ?"

"Sheila, there must be 12,000 people in here and I'll bet you're the only person focused more on the organ music than the fact that one of our guys is going to get a penalty for fighting," I said to her, laughing. And I was processing the fact that her experience of the hockey game was absolutely consistent with her own interests and life context. It was a great reminder to avoid assumptions about the other person's perspective. She was further delighted when, as the fight was ending and penalties assessed, the organist serenaded us with "Hit the Road, Jack" as the opposing player went to the penalty box.

At the first intermission (don't ask me about my attempts to explain why, in ice hockey, it is indeed called intermission, "Yes, Sheila just like at the symphony"—set me back quite a bit in my quest to get her used to "halftime" references in other sports), we went for a stroll to find the organist.

Sheila's regard for ice hockey had increased immeasurably by this discovery of live organ music to accompany the action. She wanted to know if the organist used music and was totally impressed by the repertoire needed to provide entertainment throughout an unpredictable hockey game. We actually stood and watched the organist in action for a while as the second period of the game began. I have never done that since at a hockey game and likely will not ever do it again, but I do think of her every time I hear organ music at the ice arena.

Challenges

During the winter of 2003-2004, Sheila mentioned that she was going to an appointment with her gynecologist that was outside of her usual annual check-up schedule. She explained that she occasionally was bleeding and wanted to get it checked out. When I got home on the day of her appointment, she reported that the doctor had done a biopsy ("It *REALLY* hurt") and that results would take several days. She said the doctor was not overly concerned, but thought the biopsy would rule some things out.

I was not thinking about those test results when Sheila met me in the kitchen as I came through the door several days later. "Come and sit down," she said. "I have something to tell you. There is no emergency. Don't be alarmed."

Her demeanor was not overly tense, nor did she seem particularly anxious. I thought she had received some news about a friend or maybe someone in my family back in Pennsylvania.

"The doctor called today. I have cancer."

I couldn't speak. I looked right into her eyes to read her emotions and to be sure I heard her correctly. She gave me a small nod, and said, "No matter what happens with this, I'm going to be okay. Either way, I will be fine."

Either way? She was thinking about her death? My mind was racing now, having comprehended what she was telling me.

"Sheila, did the doctor give you reason to think that your condition is not treatable?"

"Oh, no. But I want you to be sure to know that I will be fine no matter what happens. That's how I'm looking at this."

"What exactly did the doctor say?"

"There was malignancy in the cells they sampled and she's referring me to a gynecological oncologist. The office will call me when an appointment is set up. I don't know what to expect yet, other than that I will likely have a hysterectomy. That much is clear."

She was watching me closely, trying to read my expression as much as I was trying to read hers, I think. We didn't say anything at all for a few moments. Then I took her hand and said, "Sheila, no matter what, I will be in this with you. I will not back away or get scared or bail out if it gets hard. I will take my cues from you. I will do whatever you ask of me as we deal with this."

"Well," she said, standing up on her way to resume the usual end-of-day process of preparing dinner, "the first thing is, please don't treat me like I'm sick. The worst thing would be for you to pity me or feel sorry for me. Let's try to have as normal a life as possible around here. I hope that doctor appointment is soon so we can get on with this."

This was classic Sheila—to assess a situation, decide what to do, and get on with it. But I privately doubted my ability to do what I promised her I would do. I was uncomfortable with medical things, inexperienced at working through major challenges with another person, and uncertain of my own strength for what might come. Nonetheless, I resolved to do the very best I could. She was my closest friend. We depended on each other and I wanted to show her that she could count on me.

The appointment was for several weeks later making the wait for more information and a treatment plan difficult. I regularly reminded myself to act normal, per Sheila's request. But my thoughts were not normal and I could see signs of worry on her face. But we did maintain our usual routines and Sheila told only select people about her diagnosis. She invited me and her daughter Connie to come along to the appointment so there would be additional listeners to absorb the information the doctor would provide. Sheila had experience in this, having learned from Allan's illness. She asked me to take a note pad to write things down so we could review it all after the appointment. With notebook in hand and Connie in the back seat, I drove the three of us to the appointment, just twenty minutes away.

After check-in procedures were completed, an office staff member explained that the doctor would first examine Sheila and talk with her. Connie and I would be invited to join them in the doctor's office afterwards. Because patience is not my finest virtue, the wait while Sheila was in with the doctor seemed to take forever. I pretended to be reading, but could not comprehend anything on the page. I read the same page in a magazine at least four times and still didn't have any idea what was on it. I kept thinking about how much I wanted Sheila to like this doctor. My mind was busy trying to prepare intelligent questions to ask, reminding myself to take the notes Sheila wanted, and telling myself to defer to Sheila and Connie. I did not have the lead in managing this situation.

We were finally ushered into the office of Dr. David Cohn, a personable, very professional man likely in his forties. After brief introductions, he sat down behind his desk. Sheila and Connie were seated directly across from him. I was to his right with my chair perpendicular to his desk. A nurse was standing to my right.

Dr. Cohn began by reviewing Sheila's biopsy results. He spoke in detail about the kind of endometrial cancer she had, the benefits of her early diagnosis, and the need for a complete hysterectomy procedure that would also include sampling of abdominal lymph nodes. He accompanied this recommendation with a diagram he drew on a piece of paper to show the location of the lymph nodes while explaining the importance of the samples to determine whether the cancer had spread beyond the uterus.

He was the best communicator of complex, frightening information that I had ever heard. And I liked that he was making recommendations. His was not a process of presenting options and then asking Sheila to decide. I could tell she was doing fine with this fellow. He was compassionate, invited questions, seemed to be in no rush at all despite a waiting room full of people, and expressed confidence that his treatment plan would prove to be successful. The phrase I heard and held on to was, "If you have to have cancer, this is the kind to get." I even wrote it down.

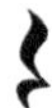

Sheila came through the surgery at the Ohio State University Arthur James Cancer Hospital with no complications. After several days in the hospital, she was discharged to complete her recovery at home. Within a week, however, came word from the doctor's office that one of twenty-two lymph nodes had tested positive for malignancy. Dr. Cohn's office recommended that an appointment be scheduled for several weeks out, to allow Sheila time to more fully recover from the surgery. At that time, a treatment approach would be discussed. The illusion that the surgery would fix the problem had vanished and now we were trying not to anticipate trouble before we had facts. The elusive ability to be patient was a challenge for both of us.

This time, just Sheila and I went to the appointment because her children's schedules prevented them from joining us.

The process was the same. Dr. Cohn spent time with his patient before I was invited into his office for conversation (with notebook in hand, per instructions from my housemate). Again, Dr. Cohn reviewed test results, discussed options, and made a recommendation that Sheila begin chemotherapy at once. We also began our journey of understanding the CA 125 test that becomes a harbinger of morale for cancer patients. At least it did for mine.

Before we left the office, we were referred to a very direct yet compassionate nurse whose job it was to explain the realities of chemotherapy to us. She provided literature to read ("I know this will be hard to remember"), a remark to which I tried very hard not to take exception as I scribbled in my little notebook. She looked straight at Sheila and said, "You will lose your hair. Not some of it, or a little bit, all of it. Some patients want to deny that. I'm telling you it will happen. Accept it as part of your treatment and healing. I will provide contacts to get a wig. Don't wait. Go do it now. It takes several weeks to get one. If you wait until you lose your hair, you won't have your wig when you need it."

She explained how chemotherapy would weaken Sheila's immune system, so it would be wise especially to avoid surfaces likely to be germ-laden (salad bars, grocery carts, door handles in public places) and suggested that we get a container of antibacterial wipes to keep in the car.

She talked about monitoring blood counts, controlling nausea, feeling the worst three days after a treatment, and unpredictable side effects that would be managed as the treatments went along.

This nurse had a way of communicating the impending discomforts and realities yet spoke with optimism about the helpfulness of the treatments. She told Sheila to keep her life going, to keep doing things she wanted to do as she felt stronger, and to not become a slave to the chemotherapy treatments—every three weeks until six treatments had been completed.

On the way home, my "take charge and face realities" friend expressed her disappointment that it was too late in the day to use her cell phone to call the wig salon to make an appointment because they were closed. I was struggling mentally trying to control increasing anxiety about my ability to provide meaningful support to someone in chemotherapy while fulfilling her repeated wish that I not treat her like she's sick.

In addition to the instructions on practical preparations, we left the office with several prescriptions and a page-and-a-half of instructions on when to take them. Sheila asked me to help her organize the medications so there was a double-check that she had it right. This regimen was important for controlling the nausea and other side effects that are all too common in chemotherapy patients.

I wasn't there for the first treatment, which was administered in the doctor's office.

Connie and her brother Mark went with their mother for her first treatment. While I felt uncomfortable being on the outside of this vital process, I understood the importance of my deferring to her children because I knew it meant a lot to Sheila to feel their interest and support. I left the office as early as possible that day, eager to hear a full report from the patient.

Sheila was eager to tell me all about it, describing the comfortable room in which the IVs were administered, the efficiency and warmth of the nurses, and brief stop-by from Dr. Cohn who said something charming to the chemo room patients (about four at a time), and of course told me all about what she learned from the other patients in the room.

I had no idea how chemotherapy is administered, so it was news to me that several people are seated in luxurious reclining chairs with snacks, books, and television available to make them comfortable. The process takes several hours, so conversation is common, a welcome revelation to my extrovert friend. I should have known that I would hear more about the condition of the woman in the next chair who was on her fourth treatment and the woman who didn't want to talk to anyone than I did about how Sheila felt. She expressed her hope that the silent one would be there again next time so she could try to learn more about her. "I hope she's not sad and lonely. It would be awful to feel that way and have cancer, too."

Sheila was herself for the next few days but did begin to drag on the third day, just as foretold by the doctor's office. She described it as feeling like she had the flu. She was tired and achy but had no trouble with nausea at all and announced that, "If this is as bad as it's going to be, it's no problem."

One weekend day after her second treatment and after she recovered from the third-day dreariness, Sheila called me into her room where she stood with her hairbrush in her hand.

"Look at this. This happened yesterday, too," she said, holding up a handful of hair. "And look at my pillow. There is hair all over the place. Will you cut my hair off for me? I don't want to find it everywhere. It's making a mess. If it's going to be lost, I want to control how this goes and get started on wearing my wig."

"Sheila, are you sure you want me to do that?" I was buying time to get myself ready for her hair loss and testing to see if she was really committed to this proposal.

"Yes!" She was emphatic. "I have to accept that this is happening. I don't want it to fall out gradually. It's clearly time for me to start getting used to wearing the wig. I really want you to cut my hair off." She was calm and matter-of-fact, in her "let's get on with it" mode.

Unsettled by this new reality and feeling honored to be asked to do this, I went for the scissors, while trying to determine if I should resist this plan so we wouldn't do something regrettable and irreversible. Once I reconciled that while this was an unusual request, it was not an unreasonable one—we stood in Sheila's bathroom that fine Saturday afternoon in April and I cut her hair off. With the trash can full and the sink a mess, we looked in the mirror and laughed at what we had just done. Clearly we were in new territory, but at least we were in it together.

Sheila got her wig out of her closet and began fussing with it. She had a streak of vanity that she acknowledged and fought with herself about. In this case, I think it was useful. When she had picked up the wig about a week prior to this, she had been pleased by the color and style, both quite similar to her usual look. Now, she worked to get herself comfortable with the reality of her new hair care.

I hung around and teased her gently about her new look, trying to smooth the transition and encourage her. She soon had her new hair looking just how she wanted it to and she was ready to move on. The only wig issue was the period of itchiness that ensued until her last little hair ends fell out, which happened in a matter of days.

Sheila tolerated her chemotherapy treatments well. I usually either took her or picked her up, sharing these support duties with two of her children. We got used to the regular routine of medications and her days of feeling unwell, trying to take to heart the nurse's encouragement to keep living while receiving the treatments.

Trouble began after the fourth treatment.

Sheila complained about pain in her leg. She had been encouraged to call at any time during her treatment if she had questions or concerns. This message was reinforced by the exceptional staff in the office during each visit. They emphasized the importance of tending to side effects early, so major and dangerous complications could either be ruled out or treated. So Sheila called.

A diagnostic test confirmed a blood clot. Sheila went right from the test center to the hospital and called my office to tell me where she was. I don't remember who had taken her for the test, but Sheila insisted that the person return home after her admission to the hospital, never wanting to inconvenience others. She then called me at the office to update me on her situation and to ask me if I could go home and collect some things she would need for her hospital stay. "They say I'm going to be here for a few days."

Coumadin by IV was being administered to treat the clot, which was small. Sheila was highly impatient with the entire process because she didn't really feel sick. "They just come in here and draw blood every five minutes." Her tendency for overstatement came out especially when she was agitated. The doctors were soon satisfied with the progress of treatment and discharged her, with the assignment of a visiting nurse to check that she was maintaining proper blood viscosity levels.

I stayed home for the nurse's visit the next morning and was stopped in my tracks when she looked at me and said, "As we continue to monitor the patient's condition over the next several weeks, it won't be done by us visiting after these first few days. She'll have to go for tests each week and, depending on the results, she may need an injection. Are you the primary care-giver? Can you give her an injection? We would teach you how, of course."

I froze. I had prided myself on doing whatever was needed to support Sheila as she battled her cancer. But I had an aversion to needles and the prospect of giving her an injection was really unsettling for me. I couldn't think of anything to say.

Sheila rescued me. "May we have some time to think about this, please? Nancy has a very demanding work schedule and may not be available when I need an injection. We may want to involve someone else."

I looked at her gratefully because she was well aware of my needle issues. Her capacity to rescue me in the midst of her own discomfort was one reason I admired and loved her so much.

"Perhaps you have a friend who is a nurse who could do this, if necessary," the nurse suggested.

"Yes. That's a good idea. We do have some friends who are nurses. We'll think about how we want to handle this," Sheila assured the nurse, and me.

"Just let me know what you decide and then call our office so we can organize a training session with the person you choose, to be sure everything goes okay," the nurse said, apparently satisfied that we could make arrangements with someone capable.

After she left, Sheila looked at me and said, "What do you think about learning to give me an injection?"

"Sheila, it's not only about my aversion to needles. Every injection I've ever received has hurt. I don't think I can do something to you that will hurt you, even if I know it's good for you. I just hate to say this, but I don't think I can do this for you. I'm sorry. I'm so sorry."

I felt terrible, but I wanted to do what was best for her. My trying to give her an injection would not be good for either of us. I hated this weakness in myself, but decided that this was no time to be heroic. Predictably, Sheila understood. She assured me that my declining to give her injections was no problem at all.

After much discussion on not bothering busy people and not involving people whose personality or discretion would require too much extra work, I finally suggested our next-door neighbor, a retired nurse. Aggie was in her seventies and was mentally sharp. She had lived beside Sheila for more than thirty years even though the relationship was not particularly close. Sheila agreed to contact Aggie to gauge her comfort level with taking this on even though she was skeptical that Aggie would accept.

I went to the office feeling like I had done the right thing, but feeling inadequate at the same time. When I got home, Sheila was smiling. She reported that Aggie was thrilled to be asked to help. Sheila had called the visiting nurse office, confirmed a mutually satisfactory time for the next evening when the nurse planned to come anyway, and arranged a meeting for all parties involved in this care plan.

It was touching to see two nurses, a generation apart, comparing notes on the evolution of needles, but acknowledging that giving an injection is quite basic. Aggie was very intent and the young nurse very respectful with their agreeing on the procedure to follow if Sheila needed an injection. After the nurse left and Sheila thanked her profusely, I walked Aggie to our front door. "Thank you, Aggie. You are really saving me. I was not comfortable with the thought of giving Sheila an injection."

"Honey, don't you worry about it. I am honored that you asked. It's nice to feel wanted and be able to use my training again at my age. Thank you for trusting me to do this." She looked me directly in the eye to convey her sincerity.

It was a good reminder that people do like to help but sometimes need to be invited to do so. She also made me feel that something redeeming was coming out of my being a chicken about administering an injection.

Sheila responded well to the blood clot medications and then had to anticipate her final chemo treatments. She was becoming emotionally weary, as having experienced four treatments and their effects, she now knew what to expect. She continued to enjoy the company of the other patients in the treatment room, but the battle of side effects (hair loss, blood clot, sores in her mouth that made eating impossible until that was dealt with, and others) was tiring.

I was attempting to maintain the aura that we were carrying on as if nothing was amiss, but it was hard for me to watch her battle, even though she was doing it with great dignity and few complaints.

I tried to provide distraction by telling her stories of office politics or crazy customers, but felt like it wasn't enough. I walked the dog for her and occasionally cooked. But Sheila did not like to relinquish her food preparation activities. Being a cook was a key part of her identity, so when I could tell that she didn't feel up to it, I suggested take-out food instead. That was more palatable for her than my doing the cooking.

Finally, we did what we had done for eight years when one or both of us needed a mental break. We planned a trip. Sheila consulted with the doctor to be sure it would be acceptable after her treatments were over. Sheila was not comfortable going very far in case she needed her doctors, so we planned a trip to the Hocking Hills area of southeastern Ohio in the fall. It was good for both of us. A change of scenery provided a respite and time to enjoy ourselves as we often did on our travels when things had been normal.

After the final chemo Sheila then began three-month check-ups with Dr. Cohn. The visit included an examination, plenty of time to consult about how she was feeling, and the inevitable blood test to assess the level of CA 125 cancer marker. She was not complaining or unusually tense prior to the appointments, but did share that she was distracted in the days leading up to the visits and during the subsequent waiting period for the doctor's office to call with the blood test results.

She liked Dr. Cohn immensely, mostly for his reassuring demeanor and professional knowledge, but especially when he told her of his plans to learn to play the cello. During her first follow-up visit, he also told her that he had modified her chemo drugs slightly to include one with reduced likelihood of peripheral neuropathy, a common side effect of chemotherapy. He did this because he knew she was a musician whose specialty was the piano. I loved the guy, too, especially when I heard that one.

It took a long while for Sheila's hair to grow back in after the chemo. She began to be annoyed by the wig, especially as her hair was getting longer and the wig was hot and a bit itchy. But she didn't really complain, rather she anticipated the time when she could abandon the wig. She made plans to visit her hair stylist for a trim, decided on a shorter style than usual, and stepped out. Her hair did not change appreciably. It was perhaps a bit thinner, but didn't get curly or change color as happens to some people. She had great hair before chemo and it came back fine after chemo. She was pleased and happy to be moving on.

We visited Savannah, Georgia in early 2005 and Sheila had a great time planning a summer trip to New York City for the women in her family. Her daughter, two daughters-in-law, granddaughter, and step-granddaughter went to the city for a long weekend. Sheila covered most of the expenses. "I'm not sure how long I'll be around to see them enjoy some things that I doubt they'd do otherwise."

She was not at all fatalistic about her diagnosis and treatment. Sheila was good at living a full and busy life, using her many gifts with much energy. But she did perhaps display a bit more urgency about some things since her diagnosis. The trip for the "wild women" of the family was one of them. They talked about it for months afterward.

In the fall of that year, after a six-month check-up, the dreaded post-visit call came. The CA 125 levels were elevated and further testing was needed. Sheila went for a scan and a suspicious spot in her abdomen was identified. The recommendation was for radiation treatment to eradicate it.

Sheila was very brave in the face of this news which, for one thing, meant she had to abandon plans to go on a cruise with her son and daughter-in-law.

I was worried about her. This seemed like a very significant development. She told me that Dr. Cohn was optimistic that the radiation would finally knock the cancer out and she believed him. I didn't doubt him, but wondered how she could keep going with such a positive attitude and with such energy in the face of what I considered to be a set-back.

Sheila insisted on going for the initial radiological consultation alone. "None of you need to take off work to go with me. I know right where I'm going because it's the same place Allan went. You would just sit there while they work with me anyway. I'll be fine. I'll tell you all about it when you get home from the office."

She did. She liked the radiologist very much, was impressed by the treatment technology, and was glad to have such easy access to a specialty hospital like the Arthur James at OSU. She went every day for three or four weeks and was tolerating the treatments just fine. The negative in Sheila's mind was that her treatments interfered with her plans to tend to a teacher colleague who was terminally ill with pancreatic cancer and had no family other than her husband who was still working. Sheila had become one of the two care-givers and hospice volunteers who made sure someone was with this woman each day. Going to radiation appointments for her own cancer was a great inconvenience in the face of Sheila's commitment to her friend who needed her.

The only times she was dragging a bit after radiation was on the days when she encountered children who were there for treatment. Sheila's feelings about her own situation leaked out a bit when she said "It is scary to go in there each day with that huge equipment in the sterile room, thinking about what they are doing to you and hoping that it works. I can't imagine what it was like for those parents or that little girl. I hope I don't see a child in there again." But she did. And this time she was in tears telling me about an infant brought in for a radiation treatment.

That was near the end of her regimen and I could tell she was getting weary, both from the treatment visits and from the toll of her care-giving. I scheduled a day off despite Sheila's objections and we spent the day having a little outing. We went to the movies ("That score was wonderful. I'm going to order the CD"), had a nice lunch, and visited the art museum. Before Sheila, I never would have set foot in an art museum. But her enthusiasm, appreciation, and knowledge had resulted in my visiting art museums all over the world. On this day, it was especially good to get lost in beauty.

When her treatments were concluded and follow-up visits finished, the doctors were very pleased with the results. Sheila had a few radiation side effects to contend with, but she was a mostly compliant patient and did as the doctors recommended.

She also had to deal with the death of her dear friend. Again, we did what we always did when we needed a break. We planned a trip. The following spring we visited my brother and his family, as well as a long-time friend of Sheila's in the Los Angeles area. We also included the classic tourist activities there and then headed for Yosemite National Park. Sheila felt quite well during the entire trip and we were optimistic that her days of battling cancer were behind her. Follow-up visits to the doctor again stretched out to six-month intervals, the CA 125 numbers were normal, and things were looking good.

That summer, July of 2007, Sheila became unwell at a small party we were attending at the home of friends. Her digestive system was not working and she had pain in her stomach. I got her home and into bed for a rest. The pain subsided and she soon returned to eating normally again. Her fall check-up with Dr. Cohn was very good and he talked to her about increasing her intervals to one year. We both were delighted.

Then just before Thanksgiving, Sheila awakened feeling ill. I had to go to Cleveland on business during the day, but she assured me that she would be fine and had people to call if necessary. I left thinking that she had a stomach virus and would be fine in a day or two. When I got home she was still in bed and reported feeling worse. (I was frustrated with myself for not having followed up with her again later in the day.) We talked about her options and finally agreed that she needed to go to the hospital and that the best thing to do was to call the ambulance, mostly because Sheila said that the effort to get warm clothes on, go downstairs and struggle into the car felt like too much. The ambulance whisked her off to the Mt. Carmel Hospital, closest to us, and I followed shortly thereafter, calling Connie as I went.

They kept her overnight and did a scan of some kind the next day that showed a slight "blockage," they thought. Sheila began to feel better and the doctor indicated that the tests were somewhat inconclusive. Slight blockages can resolve themselves and if she was feeling better, she could go home if she promised to follow up with her primary care physician after the holiday. She promised and I brought her home.

Thanksgiving Day did not go well. Sheila was with me in Pennsylvania because this was the every-other-year that all three of her children spent the holiday with the families of their spouses. That was long-standing practice which worked well for Sheila when Allan, her parents, and in-laws were living. Now, with her being alone, she had spent several Thanksgivings with my family on the off years.

Sheila became sick several hours after the meal at my brother Bob's house. We came home to Ohio the next day, with Sheila resolving to eat very little until she had more information on her condition. She went to her primary care doctor who wanted to refer her to a gastroenterologist, but with its being the end of the year holiday time, an appointment would take some time to arrange. His office promised to work on it.

Meanwhile, Sheila scheduled another follow-up visit with Dr. Cohn in December, who listened to her about this recent stomach pain and digestive difficulty and agreed with the plan to see a gastroenterologist. Nobody at the OSU hospital was available before January either. All through the month of December, Sheila ate only coffee, juice, crackers, and occasional food "because I don't want to throw up all the time or be in pain. Christmas is coming and I have a lot to do."

I knew she was feeling terrible and that her lack of nutrition was affecting her energy. This was most telling when it was time to bake cookies. Sheila usually loved Christmas baking. We had made cookies together ever since the beginning of our common household. This year, she sat and watched while I did everything because she was busy with other preparations during the day and had almost no energy in the evening and weekends. She was also recovering from tendonitis in her foot. My friend was in bad shape and I knew it. But she was seeing her doctors and waiting for an appointment about her stomach issues. She was determined to enjoy Christmas with her family.

I went to Pennsylvania as usual to be with my family and was surprised when she called me the day before Christmas. I could hear energy in her voice as she said; "Guess what? Dr. Cohn called. My CA 125 is normal. He feels good about my condition relative to cancer. I don't have to see him for another six months. It's the best Christmas gift, isn't it?"

It was, but our relief would not last long.

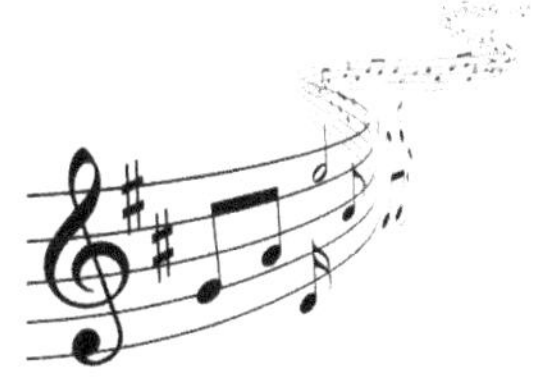

Point/Counterpoint

January 2, 2008 was the beginning of the longest and most painful year of our seventeen-year friendship. We were so full of optimism on Christmas Eve 2007 with the assurance from Dr. Cohn that a check-up appointment with him would not be needed until June. As we ushered in the New Year, we were not thinking about cancer. We were eager for a diagnosis and treatment plan to address the gastroenterology symptoms of late December 2007.

Then came the call from Sheila's primary care physician that she should come to the ER and have the gastroenterologists paged. That is when Sheila called me and I promised that I would meet her at the hospital as soon as I could get away from my office.

After I had devoted my full attention to my meeting and notified the important people that I had an emergency, I left the office early. I wanted to get to Sheila as soon as I could. I arrived at the hospital just before four o'clock and stopped at the front desk to get a room number for her. I was quite surprised and a bit annoyed when they told me she was still in the ER. I made my way impatiently through the security protocols administered by the front desk in the ER and was finally directed to Sheila's location. I was so anxious to see her.

The room was located at the far end of a wide hallway lined with various pieces of equipment and supply cupboards. There was a curtain partially drawn across the entrance to her room, which had solid walls on the sides and was comfortably sized. She heard me coming, looked up, and gave me a very weak smile.

I was disturbed by her appearance. She looked small and frail and vulnerable, not something I was used to in my strong and commanding friend. She was partially wrapped in her favorite red robe. I smiled to myself as I recognized that take-charge Sheila had taken time to pack a bag in preparation for her hospital visit, assuming that she would stay.

She was apparently cold, something unusual. She was always too warm. I was the cold one. She was all alone and feeling low, it seemed. "No wonder," I thought. "She's been in this miserable, cold ER room all alone for hours, feeling unwell, and wishing we could get on with things."

I recovered from my initial disturbed feelings and tried to put a look of optimism and strength on my face in the hope that Sheila would be fortified. She perked up a bit as we began a conversation about who her driver had been, what time they arrived, and what had occurred since. She did make me feel good when she said, "I'm so glad I have you. I knew you would come. I'm glad you're here. It's been awful just lying here all afternoon."

Not much had been going on during the afternoon, it turned out. The gastroenterologist had been paged and had ordered some tests. Results were pending. We were in the interminable waiting period. Sheila told me that she had called her three children to tell them about her need to be in the hospital that day. I don't think it would have surprised them. They knew their mother was unwell. She prided herself on preparing the Christmas Eve dinner each year. Ten days ago, she had to call them and ask that the dinner become "pot luck" because she could not manage the preparations.

I resolved to focus on Sheila, as I helped myself to a blanket from one of the cupboards in the hallway and wrapped her up so she could be warm and comfortable at least. Not long thereafter, a nurse appeared who advised that test results showed a blockage ("The doctor will come to talk to you about it soon.") and she had been ordered to insert an NG tube. This young woman exuded competence, patience, and efficiency. I felt very good about Sheila being in her care.

Neither Sheila nor I knew what an NG tube was, so this caregiver explained that it's a tube inserted through the nose, into the stomach. A pump is attached to it. In Sheila's case, the pump would be used to pump out fluids that accumulated behind the blockage, which should relieve her pain and discomfort.

"These are very difficult to insert and it is unpleasant for patients to go through. I'm sorry. This will be uncomfortable, but it will help you feel better once we get it in." she said, glancing at me and then focusing on Sheila who was listening closely. Sheila readily agreed to cooperate with the insertion of the tube.

"You will want to leave the room while we do this," the nurse said to me with a look that clearly told me not to argue with her. I really liked her take-charge attitude. "Plan to stay away for a while because this will take some time. We don't want to rush. She will be fine while you are gone. I will be sure of that," she said while uncoiling some plastic tubing from a sterile package.

"This will make her feel better," she said again as she looked directly at me. I hoped I wasn't looking skeptical or uncooperative. She clearly wanted to get on with it and wanted me out of there.

I went to the Wendy's on the same floor of the hospital, right inside the front door. I wasn't hungry, but knew that I had to eat something to sustain myself. It was after five o'clock and this was a good chance to catch my breath and get some food. The day had been a whirlwind with returning from holiday vacations, a major meeting, and the unexpected hospitalization of my closest friend.

Because I had left the office earlier than planned, I had some unfinished business to tend to. My Blackberry enabled me to do a few things while I watched the clock, trying to figure out how long to stay away from Sheila's room. It was very hard for me to focus on business problems, so I played with my Frosty (eating something I could manage to do. Eating healthy, not necessarily) and wondered what was going on in the ER. I am not good at waiting, but I was learning that medical procedures require adaptation to avoid complete meltdowns. After about twenty-five minutes, I headed back to the ER.

The curtain was completely drawn this time. "Sheila?"

"Come in. We're finished," she said immediately. I was relieved to hear her voice and to be able to get in there with her.

The nurse was standing bedside, fiddling with the newly-inserted device. Sheila was in the same position as when I left, only this time with a tube in her nose and tears trickling from her eyes. She dabbed the tears with a tissue and looked at me with weary eyes.

"I'm so glad that's over with for you," I said, trying to be positive. "It looks like you did just fine."

"She did great," the nurse said. "She is so easy to work with. Some patients fight it. She followed instructions just as I gave them and it made the whole thing go better. Now that it's in, the device will start to help."

"I sure hope so." Sheila said. "That was awful." Her tears were over and she was relaxing a bit. "I never want to go through that again."

I tried to hold on to the thought that this thing would help her. But it was hard to keep my positive face on while thinking that having a tube jammed down your throat, even by a compassionate nurse, would indeed be a dreadful experience.

"The doctor will be in after a while to talk to you," the nurse said as she patted Sheila reassuringly. "I know that was uncomfortable, but you should begin to feel better now." And off she went.

I began a monologue about the wonders of having a Wendy's in the hospital lobby and how nice it was to have a Frosty in the hope that Sheila would benefit from some distraction. We talked about inconsequential things until I thought she was relaxed enough to be practical for a moment.

"Sheila, do you want me to notify your friends that you're here?"

"Yes, but don't give them all the gory details. And tell them not to come in here. I don't need everyone to see me like this. When you're sick enough to be in the hospital, you should not have to entertain visitors."

"Right. Did you have time to prepare the distribution list in your e-mail? I am happy to keep your friends updated on your progress, but taking phone calls in the evening is not the best way to do it, especially with the number of friends you have and all of our church friends being interested in how you are doing."

Sheila assured me that there was a distribution list in her AOL address book titled "Friends and Family." She gave me her password so I could access her e-mail account. I was so glad she had done that. So many people loved her and would want to know how she was doing. It was an overwhelming thought for me, envisioning unending phone calls. I resolved to keep them all updated faithfully via e-mail.

We continued light conversation for another hour or so until a slight young woman appeared and introduced herself as the gastroenterology resident on call. She explained that a scan detected a blockage, which can be tricky to treat. Sometimes they resolve themselves. Sometimes surgery is required to relieve them. In any case, the immediate plan was to admit Sheila to the hospital to monitor her condition for several days. We were both glad for an initial diagnosis and treatment plan. Sheila was relaxing a bit and did report that she was feeling a bit better, so "it might be worth it to have gone through that draconian process."

I glanced at the beaker hanging on the wall behind her and saw an accumulation of bile-like fluid that was being pumped out of her stomach. I wondered how she was going to regain her strength. I kept trying to remind myself to keep a look of calm and optimism on my face.

I stayed with Sheila until they moved her to a private room on the ninth floor. By the time this transfer was finished and Sheila was settled in her new quarters, it was after eight o'clock. She began to fuss at me about getting home to feed the dog (of all things!) and to get some rest. She also gave me a short to-do list of things that were important to do that she had not accomplished before she left the house earlier in the day. This included mailing several greeting cards to friends, cancelling a dental appointment for later in the week, and moving some food from the fridge to the freezer. I found it reassuring to hear her give these assignments.

She did look tired, so after I was sure that she would be reasonably comfortable, I left with assurances to Sheila that I would be back the next day on my way home from the office.

The ride home was lonely. It was a dark, cold January night and the house would be empty of the usual warmth when I got home. I began my mental list of things to do when I got home in addition to those Sheila provided. Get the mail, tend to the thermostat, draw the shades, clean the cats' litter box, and write to her friends.

It had been a long day. This is what I wrote to the group under the title "**Sheila Update from Nancy**" so her friends would know who was writing to them using her e-mail.

1-2-08

Sheila asked me to let you all know that she was admitted to the hospital today for treatment of the intestinal problems she's been having. Her family doctor finally consulted with the gastroenterologist who suggested that she go to the ER and have him paged. She is in Mt. Carmel West.

After a very long day of additional tests, it was determined that she has a "high grade" blockage in her small intestine. The treatment plan is to try the least invasive procedures to resolve it. So she now has an NG tube inserted through her nose into her stomach to relieve the pressure that built up around this blockage. In some cases, the blockage is relieved after the pressure subsides and that's that.

If the tube process does not relieve the blockage, surgery may be needed. We don't know how long they will keep the tube in or when additional decisions will be made.

I know that Sheila appreciates prayers and cards, so please apply both liberally! I will update you as the situation unfolds. Hopefully, you'll be hearing from the patient herself soon. Thanks for your support and understanding of the situation.

When I arrived the next day, Sheila was sitting up in the bed and looked much better. She had an IV pole with multiple bags of medicines hanging from it. She said the doctors had been in early in the morning to check on her and to explain that the IVs were being administered in order to "improve her nutritional status." I could see how that would be necessary, given her diet for the past month or so. She was not eating anything.

She had received some mail the previous day, so I had packed that into my briefcase when I left home that morning. She opened it and provided instruction about how to handle it. I thought it was important to keep her engaged in some usual activities, thus my pony express plans.

Sheila complained about only two things, if expressing slight impatience and frustration can be characterized as complaining. She hated the tube in her nose. It was irritating her throat, made talking difficult, and kept her tethered to the hospital bed.

The aides set up a bedside commode for her to use, which was working fine; other than that she had to call the staff to assist her because of the tangled mass of IV lines and the NG tube. ("I hate to bother those people every time I need to use the bathroom.")

I thought her grouchiness was a relatively good sign. She felt well enough to complain, but the constant flow from her stomach through the tube into that beaker was concerning to me. I was watching for signs that the volume was diminishing. That wasn't happening.

Sheila was also bothered by the constant traffic in and out of her room. She was located at the very end of the hall in a small private room. She reported that "someone is in and out of here all the time." When I asked for more information, she talked about blood draws, the nutritionist, orderlies who took her for an additional scan, cleaning people, and staff who responded to the IV alerts whenever they signaled the need for a refill.

Once we reviewed the events of her day, I tried to steer the conversation to something I thought she might find more positive. "I will be writing an update note to your friends," I told her. "Why not have some visitors while you're in this waiting mode. It seems like some company might help you to pass the time."

Her response to that suggestion was immediate and left no doubt about her feelings. "No. I don't want any visitors other than you and my kids (as Sheila referred to her grown children). I don't need help to pass the time. There is something going on in here all the time. I just want to get better and go home. Please tell my friends not to come in here. If they want to do something, ask them to pray for me."

On the second day after her admission, she reported that the senior surgeon, Dr. Lowell Chambers, had been in the night before to discuss her condition. He recommended surgery. Sheila said that she liked him very much and that she agreed to surgery. "Anything to get rid of the tube and get on with this." But she needed more IV fluids to improve her status before surgery would be scheduled.

I went home that evening feeling like we were making progress and with a vow to try to deliver things to that hospital room that would make things more pleasant for my friend.

1-4-08

Sheila's treatment plan has become more defined in the past 24 hours, thanks to the involvement of the senior surgeon whose staff members have been treating her. He visited her last evening and said that, in his opinion, this blockage is not likely to be relieved via the noninvasive procedures. He recommends surgery. This opinion was seconded by Sheila's family doctor after his visit with her today—and after he had reviewed all of the test results and surgeon's notes.

The surgery is not scheduled yet. The doctors recognize that Sheila's been weakened a bit due to lack of nourishment in recent weeks. So they are infusing her with various nutrients to strengthen her system prior to the operation. We do not know how long this will go on—perhaps for a week or more.

She is resting relatively comfortably (as much as is possible anyway in a hospital) and her spirits are pretty good. She requests no visitors outside of the family because of the recommendation that she rest and strengthen herself—and it is difficult for her to talk (can you imagine ?!) due to the tube in her throat that is serving multiple purposes (don't ask).

I know that she appreciates your prayers and cards, so those are most welcome. Thanks to everyone for your interest and support. I will provide additional updates when things change. In the meantime, I'll go feed the pitiful dog who is absolutely woeful without her around here. Little does she know that she's stuck with me for a while.

I developed a new daily routine, with a focus on maintaining the home front so Sheila had nothing to worry about other than getting better. I started in a new position at my company in November, so I had plenty of work to do at the office. I left home early each morning with my briefcase and a little bag of stuff for Sheila that I had packed at night before I went to bed. I took her mail, some light reading material, and a few other items she had asked for. The hospital was conveniently located on my way home, so I developed an approach to the parking garage, navigation through the campus buildings to the proper elevator, and access to Sheila's room quite efficiently. It was usually between five and six o'clock when I got there. I'd stay for at least an hour and then head home. It made for a long day, but it was how things were for us for a while.

Sheila didn't feel like reading much, so the books I took were sent home the next day. That was a sign to me of how poorly she felt. Ordinarily, reading was a pleasure for her. She hated the tube and complained that the young doctors who were monitoring her, always showed up very early in the morning. Sheila was not a morning person and they likely woke her up. This told me that the information I was getting about what they said might be murky, but no doctor was ever there during the hours I was there.

Over the weekend, Sheila prompted me to stay home and "take a break from this." My response was noncommittal so as not to agitate her, but I knew that I would go. I felt like she needed me to come. I tried to imagine what it would be like to be in the hospital for days awaiting surgery.

I thought it was important for her to hear things from me about how normal everything was at home, so she did not spend one moment worrying about not being there, as I knew would be her tendency. I was glad that her daughter Connie stopped by on Friday evening.

Sheila fussed at me about whether I was eating. I explained that I ate more at the office and had light snacks when I got home, which was the truth. She also wanted to know how her poor dog was doing.

That story was a bit less happy. After all, it was early January and dark when I got home. And I was not in the mood to entertain a dog. So I told Shelia that I could walk the dog on weekends, but do little more than give her food and water during the week. I did sometimes have her come into the house if I got home at a decent time, so she at least had a change of scenery.

Sheila again was adamant about no visitors and was very appreciative of the cards she'd been receiving. I found something in our mailbox for her every day. She took a lot of time with each card and I just sat by quietly watching her have "a little visit by mail" with the sender. It was touching.

Apparently my e-mails were being very well received. It never occurred to me that people would write back. But Sheila's in-box was loaded with responses with people thanking me and expressing concern for her. I knew I didn't have the energy to write to each one and I felt inadequate because I didn't.

Some people wrote and asked me to add others to the distribution list. I tried, but soon got bogged down in the unfamiliar workings of AOL. I became really frustrated until I finally realized that I was just going to have to ask people to share, if others wanted to know. I was getting reconciled to my limitations in dealing with this and reminded myself that doing what Sheila needed and what our household required was a priority. I hoped her friends would understand.

One reason I was weary is that the house across the street had been sold. The person who bought it was in there each night working on it, sometimes until nearly midnight. The dog heard the coming and going and barked. I was either awakened or distracted as bedtime neared. And I didn't know what to do. Dog duty was not usually my thing. I did know that Sheila was extremely diligent about her dog's barking not disturbing the neighbors. She would go to the garage, call the dog in from the yard, and settle her.

I tried that in my jammies one night, but Hildey just went right back outside through her doggie door and resumed barking after I left. I was so tired and frustrated that I was nearly in tears.

I finally put the barrier in the doggie door to confine her inside the garage which helped the neighbors, but not me. She barked until she tired herself out. And I didn't get much sleep. I had to figure out what to do. I was not consulting Sheila, that was for sure. She was already uncharacteristically peevish and anxious to "get on with this," so I was trying to focus her attention on positive things.

1-8-08

Well, I realized as I accessed Sheila's e-mail just now that many of you are writing to me and I have to tell you that I appreciate your interest and support for Sheila. Unfortunately, I'm not able to respond to most of you individually just now, but will do the best I can to keep you informed via these group notes. I'm using a group list that Sheila hurriedly created as she was going into the hospital, so if you know of anyone who is interested in information about her situation, please feel free to forward my notes on. I'm not even sure who's on the list—and I'm grouchy about AOL since it's unfamiliar to me and I can't figure out how it works quickly enough!

Anyway, I plan to tell you three things in this note: 1. How Sheila is doing; 2. Where to mail cards; 3. How things are on the home front. Let's start with the most important thing first.

The doctors have tentatively scheduled Sheila's surgery for Monday. All indications are that this blockage is a result of adhesions—

either from prior surgeries or the radiation or both. They continue to be concerned about her overall weakness due to lack of nutrition in recent weeks, so they want to continue nourishing her via intravenous fluids for these additional days. They are closely monitoring her blood to confirm progress and see positive signs. She still has the tube in her throat to suction fluids from around the blockage. And they want her to rest and build strength. She does not want to receive visitors because "they're (the medical staff, not visitors) always in here doing something to me," which is often tiring for her. I see signs of progress because one of her requests to the courier (me) from home to hospital today was for the hairbrush, hair gel, and hand mirror. They have some kind of a nifty process that enables a hospital patient to wash her hair, which prompted a declaration that "something has to be done with this hair." I thought she looked fine, but there is no arguing with a sorority girl about her hair, so the beauty aids will be in my little bag tomorrow.

I continue to recommend cards and prayers. If it's convenient for you, please feel free to send the cards here to the house. I stop by the hospital every day on my way home and take the mail, so it's easy.

The home front is an adventure. The poor dog continues to pout because her beloved mistress is not here. When I open the door in the garage to have her come into the house, she races into the family room only to discover an empty chair where she usually finds Sheila. Then she runs all over the first floor, up the steps, back to the family room, occasionally up the steps again, before finally accepting the inevitable and slumping into a heap at the bottom of the steps with her head hanging as low as it can go.

I'm supposed to keep the bird feeders filled, but I go to work in the dark and come home in the dark, so I don't know if I'm maintaining the household standard on that or not. I know I'm not doing well on the "presentation is everything" front because I'm eating leftovers directly from the dish that went from freezer to microwave rather than "serving" them on a plate. Don't tell Sheila!

Seriously, we're all doing just fine. The patient is resting relatively well, has a good attitude about her upcoming operation, appreciates all of the prayer and mail support she is receiving, and I am holding down the home front.

I will most likely not send another note unless something changes between now and Monday. I will certainly update all of you as soon as I can after the operation. Thank you again for your support. It means a lot.

We headed for the second weekend of this saga with Sheila's becoming grouchier and my getting wearier. I was really worried about her. She said the doctors were concerned about her nutritional status and overall weakness, something that didn't seem like the optimal circumstance for a person about to undergo significant surgery. She was also telling me that the surgeon was worried about the mesh in her belly. It was placed as part of a hernia repair about two years prior. But he would have to navigate through it and/or around it to relieve the blockage.

In the midst of this mess, it became obvious that little Blanche was quite ill. We knew this was coming, as she had been diagnosed with a kidney condition that is rather common in Persian cats. The only curative option was a kidney transplant, Sheila reported to me at the end of the day of their vet visit. Even Sheila, usually the soft-hearted-do-anything-necessary one, agreed that we were not going to do a kidney transplant on Blanche.

So we were watching for signs of her inevitable decline (not making it to the litter pan, vomiting). I found those signs during this week and realized what I had to do. I talked to Sheila during one of my visits and we agreed that I should take Blanche in. The vet had an appointment available for Friday evening. I drove home after work, loaded Blanche up, went to the vet's office, then drove back to the hospital.

I cried and felt sorry for myself for a while. The daily routine was really wearing on me and taking an animal to the vet for the last time is excruciating. I was worried about Sheila and so determined to provide positive support for her. I was tired and weary and sad and nearly overwhelmed. My tears had to be short-lived as I had to get it together. Sheila needed my strength. I had to find it for her.

It was a good thing that the drive to the hospital took about twenty minutes from our house. I managed to calm myself, organize the little bag for Sheila, and deliver a positive visit for her, despite the sadness we both shared about Blanche's death. We just didn't have a lot of time to dwell on it.

At last the surgery was scheduled, despite the doctor's concerns. Sheila really wanted to get on with it and I wanted to see her on the road to recovery. Her children visited over the weekend, so she had some nice interactions with them to improve her morale for a while.

1-13-08

Sheila's surgery for tomorrow has been confirmed by the doctors. It is scheduled for 1:00 p.m., although nurses and doctors alike are cautioning that the surgery schedule is a bit unpredictable due to emergencies and cancellations that may occur tomorrow.

The doctors are pleased with the improvement in her overall condition. Her nutritional status has stabilized at a level that is very good, according to the most recent test results. Sheila is uncomfortable because the tube has irritated her throat and jaw to the point of consistent pain. The medical people say this is normal and are doing everything they can to relieve it, with moderate success (my assessment). Bad news is that it will still be in there for a while after surgery—until she's able to eat a bit. The word now is that she'll be in the hospital for "at least 4-5 days" after surgery so they can be sure that her digestive system is working as it should before sending her home.

The patient's morale is pretty good. She very much appreciates the mail she's receiving and looks forward to it each day. She is weary of tubes and IVs and her surroundings, but is ready for the procedure and recovery process ("I just want to be able to eat a salad again.").

On the home front, the dog and I took a walk yesterday which did not result in any significant bonding between us (won't happen—I'm a cat person) but did at least allow us to expend some energy in a relatively constructive way. She still looks all over the place for Sheila and will be nearly uncontrollable with joy (I'm formulating my plan on how to manage the reunion.) when she sees her again, I'm sure.

Unfortunately, we had to say good-bye to little Blanche (the cat) on Friday evening when it became clear that the time had come for her to be taken to the vet for the final time. She had been suffering from a kidney disease for many months and actually lasted a bit longer than the vets had predicted. I had consulted with Sheila about it the day before and we agreed to do it. So I'm glad that such an experience is something that I could handle while Sheila focuses on getting well. We still have the other cat, Ernie, who loves the dog and does his best to keep both of us entertained.

So that's latest from our house to yours. I will provide a post-surgical update ASAP. Thank you again for your mail and prayer support. It is very sustaining.

I don't know if prayers were sustaining me. I know that Sheila really appreciated prayers. She told me that she could feel that people were praying for her and it helped her. For me, I wasn't doing much praying, but I was working at finding positive things in the midst of this terribly difficult situation. Somehow, I was able to keep going, to stay calm, and to provide what Sheila needed.

Neither of us questioned why this illness was happening and neither one of us doubted the presence of God in our lives, including during this time. On the day of surgery, I did talk to God about blessing the doctors and bringing Sheila safely through the surgery. But I don't really believe that a loving God would do anything else, so it seemed a bit arrogant to think that I was drawing God's attention to my particular concerns for the time.

It was a very early morning, as surgery days usually are. I took the day off from work and arrived at the hospital at six o'clock. I wanted to be able to see and talk to Sheila before the procedure.

Her children were all there a short while later, which pleased both of us. I mainly stayed in the background while they interacted with their mother in the surgical holding area as nurses and doctors stopped by for pre-procedure briefings.

Dr. Chambers came in and again went through his concerns, emphasizing that he could not fully predict how things would go, but would know more "once we get in there." He was careful to guarantee nothing and to create expectations for an extended period of recovery, until Sheila's digestive processes could return to normal. I was glad to have met him and felt that Sheila was in good hands with him.

It was an interminable day. I had packed a bag for myself, full of reading material and treats. I was not going to risk being out of the area when a doctor showed up, so I took my own food.

I was restless and anxious for word on how the surgery went. I felt trapped in the crowded waiting area and this increased my anxiety. As people were called to go be with their loved ones, it emptied out and felt better. But I was having a hard time waiting to hear the outcome of Sheila's procedure. I needed her to be on the way to recovery.

When we were finally notified that the procedure was over and she had come through fine, my relief was palpable. We all went to the room after she was moved there from the recovery area.

After everyone left, I stayed for a while. I didn't want to leave her, even though she didn't know I was there after a while. I just wanted to stay. So I just sat there with her as the nurses came in and out, doing the usual post-surgical monitoring. I talked to Sheila quietly, not caring if she could hear me after she settled down. If she could, I wanted her to know that I was still there with her.

It was calming to be there after a day of being in that over-populated waiting area full of tension, so I stayed for a while. It was nearly eleven o'clock when I left to go home, feed the animals, collect the mail, and write to her friends. I needed to do that before I went to bed.

1-14-08

I know it's getting late and you have probably all been anxiously waiting for me to write, but our dear patient was in surgery today for 5 hours! Wouldn't you know that Sheila would have to exceed expectations?

Sheila's son and daughter visited with her prior to the procedure (as did Pastor Ruth) and we all agreed that she looked very good and had evidently benefited from the nutritional supplements that she's been receiving. Her chief surgeon, Dr. Chambers, is very charming and thoroughly reviewed the surgical plan with her. He continued to express concern about the complexity of the procedure due to possible radiation scarring and surgical adhesions, not to mention the blockage that was the primary target of the operation to begin with. The testing could only tell the doctors so much. The true story would only be clear once they "got in there."

Everything started on time at approximately 1:00 p.m. We were directed to the surgical waiting area and discovered that there was standing room only. Monday must be a busy day for hospitals. A very kind volunteer lady ushered us into the private room usually used only for consultations with doctors—and the wait began. At just after 3:30 they called to the waiting area from the operating room to say that everything was going fine, but it would be about 90 minutes longer. By 5:30 most all families were gone and we had visited Wendy's, Tim Horton's, the vending machines, the rest rooms (multiple times), and relocated from the private room to other more suitable seating—twice. I had read my book, worked the Sunday crossword, listened to my IPod, watched some VERY bad daytime TV (briefly), read two daily newspapers, taken a walk, eaten my snacks, exhausted all reasonably polite forms of conversation, and generally lost my patience.

Finally, at nearly 6:00 p.m., the doctor called the waiting area (the nice volunteer ladies were long gone and the vending machines had been thoroughly raided) to let us know that Sheila was in the Recovery Room. He reported that, sure enough, there was quite a bit of radiation scarring, which accounted for the length of the procedure. But, according to son Mark (who took the call from the doctor), everything went well, the blockage has been relieved (don't know details about exactly what they did), and things were looking good.

Sheila was moved from the Recovery Room to her regular room at about 8:00 p.m. and the nurses were extremely attentive (she had them all charmed within two days of arriving). They got her settled, administered extra doses of pain medication, gave her extra blankets because she was cold, and assured us that she would be closely watched all night. She's connected to too many tubes and IV lines for me to describe—all apparently routine for a procedure like this. I take my cues from the nurses. They all seemed to be quite calm about everything, so that's good enough for me.

So, there is much to be thankful for. The nurses told me they will get Sheila up tomorrow (hard to imagine, but it's apparently a good thing) and then the process of reintroducing food to her system will begin sometime after that.

On the home front, the dog was thrilled to see me come home. I think she had given up on the possibility of receiving dinner today, so I was a real hero! Ernie, in typical cat fashion, expresses little enthusiasm one way or the other about my comings and goings. As for me, I'm extraordinarily glad that Sheila has come through this operation and can now focus on achieving a full recovery.

I will continue to keep you updated via e-mail and will try to provide additional information after someone has more conversation with the doctors. Thank you again for your mail support and prayers.

I was very anxious to see Sheila the next day, so left the office earlier than usual for my hospital stop. Again, I was laden with cards from the day before and full of anticipation as I walked into her room.

To my amazement, Sheila was sitting up with the tray table pulled across the bed in front of her. She had a pencil in her hand and a small writing tablet in front of her. I was so happy to see her so well. Connie was seated at the foot of the bed.

"Wow. You look wonderful," I said to Sheila and looked into her eyes to see what there was to see. Before I was through assessing that, she said. "Don't be too happy. Dr. Chambers was here this morning. I have stomach cancer."

I stared at her and desperately tried to control my reaction while being sure I heard her correctly.

"Sheila, what did you say?" My thoughts became a blur. This made no sense. They hadn't even operated on her stomach. Was she in a morning stupor when a doctor came by? Had she been dreaming? The test results from Dr. Cohn did not indicate any reason to worry about cancer. All of these thoughts were racing through my mind as she said again, "I have stomach cancer."

I glanced at Connie who gave me a small "Beats me, I guess we have to believe her" shrug as I wondered how she could look so calm. I then directed my attention back to Sheila. "Exactly what did the doctor say? And which doctor was here?"

She was going to be annoyed with my need to analyze, I could see. But she said, "Dr. Chambers came in and told me himself this morning. They are going to do some tests, but he's quite sure I have cancer. So we have some plans to make. First of all, don't you tell anyone. I don't want them all thinking this is a death sentence and feeling sorry for me. Just don't tell anyone. I'll tell Mark and Allan (her sons) and that's it."

Egad, what plans was she determined to make less than 24 hours after a major surgery and in the face of this news? She was clearly in take-charge mode and it was pointless to resist. My mind was reeling, so I decided to stop probing Sheila and sit down.

Now, the happiness I felt seeing her sitting up and conversing so freely was just destroyed by what she was saying. I still doubted that she understood correctly. But she seemed so sure. And I was rattled.

Sheila then turned her attention to Connie and began giving her a to-do list that included plans to take over Sheila's check book. "She might as well get used to it," she explained to me later. "She is my power of attorney for business affairs."

"Good lord, Sheila," I thought. "I'm still digesting this news and you're giving instructions to your POA!" I realized that it was not helpful to argue with her and I tried to turn my attention to something constructive, but had a hard time finding anything other than the mail. This was such crushing news. I wondered how long my resolve to be positive would hold up.

On the way home, I began to consider how to write to the e-mail friends. I didn't want to lie, but couldn't tell the whole truth without impeaching on the wishes of my dearest friend who was quite clear about what she intended.

1-15-08

Just a quick note to let you know that Sheila's post-surgical activities—doctor visits, tests, nursing care, grogginess, pain, and drainage tubes, are all underway and apparently going well. I was amazed to find her sitting up in bed visiting with her daughter Connie when I arrived at the hospital about 5:00 p.m. today. She's receiving pain medication and is very tired, but is better than I thought she would be.

Sheila reports that she spent two hours sitting in her chair today, which is remarkable to me. The doctors visited with her, and she's receiving wonderful care from the nurses. So I'm not likely to send an update for several days, until after there is more to report.

Thanks again for your support. It is very much appreciated.

Sheila had been in the hospital for fifteen days and in that time I learned that the heroes of health care in hospitals are the PCAs (personal care assistants). They are low in the pecking order and have the messiest responsibilities. They clean up the vomit, administer the baths, empty the bedpans, and escort patients through their bathroom processes. Each and every one who attended to Sheila loved her while being thorough and positive with her. Sheila, of course, knew them all by name and had learned pertinent details of their personal lives and professional aspirations.

Two of them were tending to her in the bathroom when I arrived on the second day after surgery. I remember thinking that it seemed early for Sheila to be walking to the bathroom, what with a major abdominal incision, and soon learned that this circumstance was exceptional.

Sheila heard me come into her room and called from the bathroom, "This is humiliating! They've given me Lasix (a powerful diuretic) and I have to go to the bathroom all the time. I can't get here in time and I've had accidents that these girls have to clean up. I don't understand why they would do this to me." She was near tears and as distressed as I had ever heard her. Her distress set me instantly on high alert.

I tried to control my anger. Clearly, someone had to advocate for the patient. I knew that the PCAs were not the people to talk to and they were busy tending to Sheila anyway. They were moving her back toward to bed as I stood there trying to quickly determine my options. I was unfamiliar with hospital procedures, a source of frustration, especially now.

When Sheila was settled back in the bed (with a pronouncement that she would not be there long because the medicine was clearly working to flush fluids from her system), I followed one of the PCAs out of the room and said, "This is not a good situation. If this were your mother, what would you do?"

"I'd call for her nurse. But don't tell her I said that. We're not supposed to say these things. But this lady is very nice and she can't help it. The doctor should do something. Do you want me to call her nurse?" I loved that little (because she was short in stature, not little in character) PCA more than usual at that moment and assured her that I would not rat her out.

While I waited for the nurse to arrive, I could see that talking to Sheila at any length was not going to happen. She was uncomfortable and busy tending to the demands of her condition. I was in her room long enough to assure her that I was going to talk to the nurse to request an adjustment to her treatment. She expressed skepticism that I could make anything happen, which made me all the more determined.

I waited in the hallway after making a call to the home of our handbell director to explain that I was detained at the hospital with Sheila, and my arrival at practice very uncertain. (Yes, I know that musicians call it rehearsal. But I'm the athlete, remember.)

To her enduring credit, Margie simply said; "I understand, Nancy. Don't worry about it. You stay there as long as you need to. We'll do the best we can without you. It's more important that you be there if Sheila needs you there. Tell her we are praying for her." She gave me a great gift that evening, responding that way. I had one less thing to worry about at a time when that was exactly what I needed.

When the nurse arrived, I introduced myself as having Sheila's medical POA. I didn't even remember if that was true, but I was claiming it for this evening. If they asked me for proof, I would deal with that later. Sheila and I had talked about all of that when we got our legal affairs in order, but I honestly didn't remember what she had decided.

Even so, tonight I was going to get something done and thought this was the best way to get the nurse's attention. If it didn't work, I had already decided I would call Connie and ask her to produce whatever paperwork was needed along with whoever had to make a decision.

"Who are you?" she asked showing what I took to be annoyance. This one did not exude the warmth and compassion that I would have hoped. I resolved to make my request as politely as possible despite my increasing fury over this entire situation.

"I'm her housemate and medical POA. She had abdominal surgery less than 48 hours ago and has apparently been administered

Lasix. She does not have a catheter. If she needs Lasix, it seems like she needs a catheter. She cannot get in and out of bed repeatedly without exhausting herself or causing damage or both. Can you please consult with the doctor about this concern?"

She studied me ever so briefly as I plastered a look of determination and respect, I hoped, on my face.

"Yes, I will contact the doctor, but I don't know what he'll say." And off she went. I went back into Sheila's room long enough to tell her that the nurse was going to consult with Dr. Chambers in the hope that some adjustment could be made. I suggested that a catheter would be a good option. Sheila immediately reacted with resistance until I pointed out that it was too late to change the medicine that she'd already been given. We had to deal with the effect it was having on her. I tried to be brief and logical.

Sheila was clearly becoming exhausted from the ordeal of the evening. One of the PCAs was hovering nearby and jumped in to assist as Sheila announced a need to use the bathroom again. I stepped out into the hall and tried to find something redeeming in this visit.

About an hour later, the nurse came down the hall and told me that the doctor ordered a catheter for Sheila. She also looked more annoyed this time, especially when she said, "Dr. Chambers said I should apologize for this. She never should have been given the medicine after the post-surgical catheter was removed. It was an oversight. I'll send someone down to get the catheter in."

I didn't care if she was annoyed. I only cared that Sheila's situation was being improved. I did wonder if anyone on the staff would have called if I had not come in that evening. How long would the nurse in charge allow her patient to suffer like this? Surely training would tell a nurse that something was wrong. Would anyone have taken initiative for a patient without an advocate present?

I stayed until the person came to get the catheter set up. Sheila was tired and testy and completely out of sorts. I was tired and hungry and thoroughly discouraged about what was happening. This was not positive progress and we'd had no time to talk more about the cancer findings. I was getting very frustrated by lack of contact with the doctor.

I was sad and discouraged on the drive home. I felt bad about missing handbell practice despite Margie's assurance that it wasn't a problem. I knew very well that it was. Handbell ringing is a highly interdependent endeavor and it's a mess when someone wipes out at the last minute. It was also therapeutic for me to go there and make music for an hour each week. It demanded my undivided attention, a welcome island of beautiful production in a sea of uncertainty and frustration.

I didn't want to deal with an excited dog or well-intentioned phone calls or any household necessities. I wanted to be confident that Sheila's night would be better than her evening, but I wouldn't know that until the next day. I was really low. And it was snowing to beat the band, so it was a long, tense drive home.

The next day was better, thank goodness. I arrived to find Sheila propped up in bed, reporting that the catheter had helped her settle for the night. She still seemed rather listless, but she did seem to perk up as our visit progressed. I was taking mail every day (only cards now. I decided that bills would pile up at home until later.), and she became much more animated when reviewing her mail. She had wonderful friends.

I was not learning much about her condition. She didn't have more information about the cancer. She did say that the doctor told her that she would be referred back to Dr. Cohn for consultation, but the first priority was to get her digestive system working again. That was the sole focus for the moment. I guessed we'd go with that, then.

1-18-08

Our patient has had two pretty good days and one lousy day since I last wrote. Overall, she is making steady progress. She continues to be weak, sore, and tethered to various tubes, IVs, oxygen, and a self-administering pain medication machine (one of modern medicine's excellent inventions, if you ask me).

More details about the surgical procedure are gradually unfolding. Remember, the primary source of information at this point is the semi-groggy patient herself, who is having conversations with doctors who visit as early as 6:00 a.m. And you know that Sheila is not much of a morning person to begin with, not to mention being three days removed from major abdominal surgery. Anyway, they had to perform a resection of her intestine rather than simply removing the adhesion. This was an option all along, but is the most serious approach to relieving the obstruction. So her recovery will take longer, as I understand it. The current plan is to continue to strengthen her. She is receiving various nutrients intravenously as well as the usual post-surgical antibiotics and whatever else is hanging from that IV pole (**lots** of stuff).

Today, she took several walks as ordered by the doctors. The nursing and personal care staff assist her and are encouraging. But this is a significant effort and very tiring. She is still not receiving any food or liquids outside of the IV fluids. The doctor explains that starting to eat clear liquids is still several days away. So I assume that she will remain in the hospital for a while longer since she will not be released until after she tolerates real food (again, this is the way I understand the plan).

Sheila's morale is pretty good. She is enormously touched and heartened by the cards she is receiving. Thank you so much for remembering her. She is so pleased when I arrive with the mail each day. "Oh, the mail. This is the highlight of my day." (And I would have thought that my smiling face would be the topper!)

I can see flashes of Sheila's personality even through the haze of her recovery efforts. I told her I thought she looked good one day this week—and I meant it. Her immediate reply: "Well, it's dark in here." Another day I prompted her to use the little breathing machine that all surgical patients have. After about four breaths, she stopped and said, "I wonder what embouchure to use with this? I think maybe French would be best." EGAD! (Only musicians will get it immediately. The rest of you will have to look it up.)

On the home front, Ernie the cat, Hildey the dog, and I are doing fine. We don't eat as well as we do when the cook is here, but none of us lack nourishment. The dog has stopped running all over the house looking for Sheila and has instead resorted to trying to engage me in some form of dog play. (I want to say to her, "Remember, I'm a cat person.) I'm mostly not interested, but do occasionally try to participate just so she's not completely in the dumper by the time Sheila gets home. I am having some success teaching her how to watch Columbus Blue Jackets hockey games. But she usually falls asleep and I'm on my own with that—come to think of it, it's just like what Sheila does!

Sheila continues to request no visitors outside of the family. Again, I thank you for your cards and prayers. She is very much sustained by both from everyone and will continue to need both for some time.

I hope all of you are well. I appreciate your notes to me and your understanding that I'm unable to respond individually to each of you. I will write again in a few days to report on progress.

There was little evidence of consistent recovery and I was getting scared. Sheila had been in the hospital for nearly three weeks and she actually seemed worse on some days. She was sleeping a lot and still had tubes connecting her to her hospital bed. She sometimes didn't even rally much when I arrived. I tried to ask her what the doctors were saying, but she relayed confusing information from day to day.

I thought she should be feeling better more than a week after her operation. Sheila's son Mark and her granddaughter Claire visited over the weekend and were not overly alarmed. But Sheila was becoming disengaged from what was happening. I wanted to fight for her so I decided to do something. But I didn't know quite what to do. Again, my lack of experience and knowledge of hospital matters was frustrating.

I formulated a plan to involve the family doctor. He had been coming in to see Sheila every few days. I was sure that Connie knew him and just as sure that I didn't. Thus, I decided to call Connie to ask her to contact him. I wanted her to ask for his assessment of Sheila's condition so we could determine if something should be happening that wasn't. I felt better after discussing the lack of progress with someone in the family and about getting some direct input from a physician who knew Sheila well.

The family doctor did consult with Connie, but was deferential to Dr. Chambers while expressing no undue concern about Sheila's condition. This was clearly troubling—if not unbelievable—to me. Was I the only one who could see how much she was unlike herself?

I then felt better when Dr. Chambers himself came in while I was there over the weekend. I genuinely liked him. He was totally focused on getting Sheila's digestive system to work so she could be referred to the oncologist. He did not seem unduly concerned at the time, so that was reassuring. The nurses also talked about the fact that it takes time to get the digestive system "awakened" after a surgery like Sheila had. No one except me seemed to be distressed. I was reading all the signals from Sheila's behavior and thought that distressed was the only way anyone who saw her could be.

I became upset one day when I got to the hospital and found that Susie and her four-year-old daughter had been to visit.

"What?" I asked in alarm. "Are they not on the distribution list you made? How could they not be clear that you've requested no visitors other than family members?" By this time I was nuts. And it was convenient to have someone to be mad at.

"It's okay. They weren't really here that long. I guess they think they're family," Sheila said in her typically forgiving and tolerant way. But she was extra tired and did remind me to tell the e-mail friends that she didn't want visitors. "And don't get them all alarmed about how sick I am," she added. So my mandate to keep things light with the e-mail crowd remained intact.

What further upset me was the fact that she was too tired to visit with me that evening and I resented it. I wanted and needed to talk to her. I missed our daily talks at the end of the day. I was astounded that someone would disregard the specific wishes of someone in the hospital and come to visit anyway.

It was hard for me to feel very good about things on the way home that day. I was really missing Sheila's presence at home since, prior to her hospitalization, our household routines had evolved to a nice comfort level of shared responsibilities.

With her out of commission for so long, I was struggling with my new job, the animals, visits at the hospital, and running our household alone. And I felt the burden of the secret I was carrying about cancer being part of our lives again.

I didn't realize how overwhelmed I was feeling until I decided to call my friends David and Lisa for help at the house. I knew that Lisa could help me with kitchen things and that David could handle some overdue household chores that I just had not gotten to. They had repeatedly offered to do anything we needed and I was ready to ask. I was home early from an off-site meeting on a weekday and dialed their number, expecting to leave a message because they would still be working. To my surprise, Lisa answered the phone.

"Lisa, I'm calling because I need help. Can you and David come over this weekend and help me do some things around here?"

"Of course," she replied. "How is Sheila doing?" She quickly added that she was home that day due to a modified teacher day schedule.

I started my answer and could not speak. Tears poured from my eyes and I couldn't stop them. I tried to answer her. "She's not getting better," I sobbed into the phone. "I'm so scared. She's not getting better. She should be getting better by now." I cried and cried and cried at the sound of my friend's willingness to help and her concern for Sheila. It all came pouring out of me at that moment.

And my precious friend's response was perfect. She didn't say a word. She just listened to me cry until I was all cried out. And then we made plans for them to come help me.

Lisa may or may not have known that her presence on the end of that phone was a much-needed outlet that day. In the midst of this saga I was living through, I viewed this as a gift from a friend who knew how to be a friend and how to act like we're supposed to act if we pay attention in church each week.

1-22-08

Our patient has had several pretty good days. Her morale sagged a bit over the weekend one day when it seemed to her like there is no end in sight to this ordeal, but she rallied in the last two days and is feeling better emotionally now, I think. Some of that is due to some small progress in her physical condition. The doctors have removed the NG tube and oxygen, so Sheila is tethered to fewer devices than she has been. Even though it's an extreme effort, she is taking several short hallway walks each day, aided by the personal care staff. She is not yet able to do that herself, mostly because of the extreme soreness in her belly from the incision and amount of manipulation which occurred to her intestines during the operation.

I was present when the doctor visited over the weekend and he explained that they are withholding food because they want the resectioned part of her small intestine to heal before introducing food. So she still has not received any liquids or food by mouth and apparently won't for a little while yet. Sheila told me that the doctor visited today and reiterated this and reminded her that, the longer the operation, the longer it takes to restore some basic functionality in the digestive system. Since her procedure was more than five hours long, it will take a while, it seems. So there is no discussion yet about her coming home.

Sheila continues to request <u>no visitors</u>. She is expending considerable energy to do the basic things needed to aid her recovery and says that visits would be too much for her to handle at this time. I know that she appreciates the cards. When I left today, she reminded me to be sure to bring the mail tomorrow. With the holiday, it's been several days since she's received those expressions of love and concern from all of you and I think she's missed them. So I'll deliver as many of those as you can send!!

On the home front, the dog and I took several walks over the three-day weekend even though we nearly froze. I can tell you that I learned about the extreme precision involved for a dog when selecting an appropriate location to do her "business." I have never seen such sniffing and semi-squatting, and relocating and circling and revisiting the same territory in search of an exact location for elimination! It feels silly to stand there watching such activities. And just in case you canine lovers out there think I'm completely heartless, I want you to know that during those two recent nights when the temperature was in single digits, I actually gathered up the dog's bedding and put it in the dryer right before she went out so her place in the garage would be extra warm, at least for a little while. I tell Sheila that her dog is treated better than many of the children of the world—and that I am now trained to perpetuate it!

I was also reminded about the grocery store this weekend. Our usual household process is for me to handle joint finances for household bills and Sheila handles grocery shopping. After more than two weeks of her absence, the time came for me to hit the grocery store. I did just OK—had a list, located what I needed and then discovered that several things seemed to fall into my cart that were not on my list (Ben & Jerry, Cheez-its, Little Debbies). I think there's a rule that, once that happens, you have to buy them and eat them. So I did.

On the whole, we're doing OK with all of this. Thankfully, Sheila is making progress at a rate that the doctors expect. She is very much sustained by your support by mail and prayer. Her children and grandchildren are very faithful with visits that lift her spirits. We're looking forward with positive thoughts and will continue to keep you updated.

When I arrived that evening, Sheila looked especially bad. She was sleeping soundly and had difficulty getting awake to talk to me. She had always said that I should awaken her when I came to visit and I sometimes didn't. But that day, I was hoping to see progress. I was really disappointed by her appearance.

After she awoke and we had exchanged a few words, Sheila said, "I'm glad you're here. The doctor is coming this evening to talk with me about how to spend my final days. I don't know when he's coming, but he's coming this evening. I want you to hear what he says."

My stomach was instantly in knots as I tried to process this. Was this another case of confusing information because someone talked to her when she was groggy? What in the world had happened in the last 24 hours that required a conversation about Sheila's final days? I stared at her but she was weak and tired and clearly in no mood for conversation, even with me, as she put her head back on the pillow and closed her eyes. I just stood there trying to control my emotions and collect my thoughts. I told Sheila I would be right back. She nodded slightly to acknowledge that she had heard me.

I stepped out into the hall and went in search of her nurse. By now, I knew most of her care-givers by name. I wanted the nurse to review the events of the day with me so I could sort this out. I found her at the nurse's station at the other end of the hall and asked if she could spend a few moments updating me on Sheila's condition. This nurse was quite likeable, unlike the one with whom I had had the catheter war.

I explained that Sheila was relaying some information that concerned me and I wanted to understand if her condition was significantly worse. I also wanted to know if she was expecting Dr. Chambers that evening.

She told me that she was not authorized to tell me much without Sheila's permission. I pulled the "I'm the medical POA" trick out of my bag (reminding myself to try to verify that sometime soon, in case I ever really needed to prove it) and she became more willing to provide information. She told me that Sheila developed a fever during the day and was taken for a scan of some kind. She wasn't sure of the scan results, but they were administering IV antibiotics. She also could not confirm if Dr. Chambers was expected. If anyone had taken my blood pressure at that moment, I believe I might have required admission for treatment myself.

"Sheila is telling me that he's coming to talk to her about how to live her final days. Is something happening to suggest that she is in critical condition and not likely to survive?"

The nurse then told me that she could not say anything more. I would have to talk to the doctor. I was gripping the edge of the counter of the nurses' station, trying to remain civilized.

"Is there any way for you to verify that he is coming to see Sheila tonight? If he is, I need to be here. She asked me to be here. But I don't know if she understands his schedule. I don't want to wait here unnecessarily if he won't be in until sometime tomorrow." She finally agreed to contact Dr. Chambers to see if he was coming by that evening.

It was a Wednesday. I had to call Margie again and tell her that I would likely either be late for handbell practice again—or even miss it completely. I made up a story about Sheila having test results that the doctor was going to talk about and Sheila wanted me to stay for the evening. Margie's positive response was just what I needed.

I dragged a chair out from Sheila's room and sat in the hallway outside her door to wait for the doctor after the nurse had confirmed that he was coming "later this evening." Sheila was not in a condition for conversation anyway, so I sat there and worked unsuccessfully to control my anxiety. I decided not to call her children until I knew more. I wanted to believe that Sheila was confused, but had to steel myself for what the doctor might say. I tried very hard to not get ahead of myself. "Deal with the situation after you have the facts," I kept telling myself. But I could not quiet my mind.

It was more than an hour later when Dr. Chambers came down the hall. I stood to greet him and said, "Dr. Chambers, Sheila tells me you are here to talk about her final days. Is that correct?"

He stopped and looked at me briefly and said, "Please wait here. I need to see my patient privately for a moment," and moved into Sheila's room, closing the door behind him. After a few moments, he came back into the hallway and said, "Please come in. I hope you understand. I had to verify that I have permission from my patient to include you in a conversation about her." I nodded to him and followed him back into the room.

Sheila was sitting up and seemed to be alert, to my astonishment. Dr. Chambers walked around the bed and sat in a chair beside her bed while I stood on the other side of the bed with my back to the door, facing him.

He began, "Sheila, you have an infection. We are not sure of the exact cause but it is a concern. If the infection is at the site where we resected your bowel, it is very serious. It may be that there is a leak at the site where the two ends are supposed to be connected. If you don't respond to medications, our only alternative would be to do surgery to repair the leak. We know that, if a second surgery is required, fifty percent of people survive the procedure. Now, I'm saying that we do not know that you will need a second surgery, but I have to tell you what we may be facing here. That is why you had a scan today. We are trying to see what is going on in your belly. I know the scans are not pleasant, but they tell us what we need to know to treat you properly. For now, we are going to keep the antibiotics going, monitor your temperature closely, and do additional scans to watch for any signs of leakage at the resection site. The tests have been inconclusive so far. That is good." He then added, "What questions do you have?"

My heart was in my throat. A fifty percent chance of survival? Were we really heading to Sheila's "final days?" Surely not. We had too many things to do. Surely she was going to come through this and get to Dr. Cohn. Surely.

My mind was racing again even though I tried to calm myself. I don't even remember if Sheila asked a question, but I told him that Sheila was concerned about her final days.

"Oh, no," he replied. "We are a long way from that. We think we can get her through this. We are optimistic that she will respond well to the antibiotic treatments and we can get on with getting her digestive system to work. Aren't you ready for your favorite foods again?" he asked, now looking at Sheila.

With this, Sheila perked up and assumed her most charming mood. The two of them proceeded to have a light conversation about her diet and the eating habits she was anticipating.

I was still trying to absorb the fifty percent worst case scenario information. And I began to wonder what I would say to the e-mail crowd about this.

After Dr. Chambers left, Sheila was awake enough to talk with me for a while. We didn't mention the possibility of surgery. I was talking about how sure I was that she would respond to the antibiotic treatments and then get on with resuming her regular diet.

In this welcomed vein of "normal mode," Sheila complained about her ride to the place in the hospital where her scan was administered. "The ride was just abominable. It's so bumpy. Someone should do something to make it more comfortable for people in hospital beds to go get scans."

Relieved to have something this mundane in the conversation, I asked, "Sheila, what made it bumpy? These halls are nice and flat. I don't understand how the ride could be bumpy." I felt a sense of great relief to be able to focus on her and not on controlling my own panic.

"Well, it's getting into the elevator," she said like it was the most obvious thing in the world. "You have no idea how much of a bump it makes when one of these beds is pushed into an elevator. It is the worst part of the whole thing. They need to build ramps for the beds to get into the elevators," she stated with considerable conviction.

This discussion was the perfect distraction to keep me from perseverating on the fifty percent chance of survival from a possible surgery, so I stuck with it for a while, as I continued to engage her in conversation. "Sheila, that doesn't make any sense (remember, I'm a thinker according to Myers-Briggs; she's a feeler). There is no way to build a ramp into an elevator. When the door opens, the floor of the elevator is level with the floor outside in the hall. How would you build a ramp?" I really didn't get it.

"I don't know. But someone should figure it out. That ride was dreadful." She then launched into a description of the "nice young man" who was her "driver," including his entire educational history, family background, and tenure at the hospital. I was heartened at this return to her being herself.

I called Connie on the way home to relay the information on the new developments and asked her to inform her brothers. And I tried very hard not to think about the fifty percent. For once, I was almost glad to see the dog. She was a good distraction on this emotionally draining night.

1-23-08

We have a concern today. Sheila developed an infection in her abdominal area that has the doctors concerned. They are treating her with antibiotics and are hoping for a good response. If she does not respond favorably, additional surgery will be necessary. The doctor expresses great concern about this possibility because she is in a weakened condition and the surgery would be "difficult."

So let's all "pray without ceasing" that the antibiotic treatment will be effective.

I'll keep you updated.

1-24-08

The initial signs are good today regarding Sheila's response to the antibiotics to treat her infection. Her temperature is down and her white blood cell count is down. Neither has progressed as much as the doctors would like, but the trends are positive at this point. They are doing cultures to confirm the exact nature of the infection and will adjust medications depending on the results.

She continues to be very weak and gets tired easily, but her mental outlook was more positive today than yesterday when news of the infection hit. She's been in that same hospital room since January 2 so the days run together and the scenery is not very inspiring. Even positive and optimistic Sheila gets a bit blue sometimes. She continues to appreciate your cards and notes very, very much and always expresses amazement when I come in with mail every day. "I have the nicest friends," she says.

Her family doctor visited this morning. He has been extremely attentive, visiting her nearly every day. He told her that they found the infection early and that he was optimistic about her responding to the treatment. The surgeon stopped by this evening and told her that he was going to do everything he could think of to avoid additional surgery. So they are keeping an eye on her. That reassures me.

We're developing a routine on the home front. The dog is glad to see me when I come home since I'm now the food source and I'm better than nobody, I guess. I'm not as glad to see her, but we're developing an understanding of each other. Ernie the cat is generally indifferent to me unless he wants something. Typical cat attitude. We all miss Sheila very much and hope for her return home soon. Thanks again to everyone for your support to all of us, especially to Sheila. It's really helping.

It may be a few days before another update unless something changes significantly.

Prior to this new worry I felt I had regained my footing after my breakdown on the phone with Lisa. I was poised for Sheila to have surgery, recover, and get home. With this new development, I had to accept that this was going to be a very long process. I was able to adjust my expectations, something I remembered Sheila talking about from her days of being an advisor to an Alateen group in her school district: "Modify expectations so you limit your own pain when bad things happen, especially when your experience tells you that bad things are likely to happen."

I decided to help myself by focusing on Sheila and what she needed. She was the one who had been in the hospital bed for the past twenty-six days. She was the one who had undergone significant abdominal surgery. She was the one unable to eat, whose only contact with loved ones was with me and occasionally her children.

Being confined in a hospital was a terrible existence for such a social person as Sheila. I had to keep finding ways to stay positive with her. She did tell me that she looked forward to my coming each day and we were sometimes able to have our usual end of day conversations, except the topics of discussion were different. She did have some good days, so I decided that it was right to speak with her about her business affairs. I mentioned that there was mail for her at home that should be handled. She wanted me to give it to Connie, who had previously received her POA instructions.

I somehow also remembered to look into her little appointment book to see if anything had to be rescheduled. There was an endodontic appointment and a lunch date. I made those calls and suggested that we cancel rather than reschedule since Sheila's return to good health was hard to determine. I was taking my cues on this from the nursing staff. Someone usually came in during the time I was there visiting in the evening. They changed the IV bags or took blood or measured something. I asked about the long recovery time. None of them were particularly alarmed. They spoke optimistically about the patience required to work through this kind of recovery and expressed great optimism that all would be well. I was wishing I felt as confident.

1-27-08

Our patient has had several relatively good days since I last wrote. The signs that Sheila is responding to the antibiotic treatment continue to trend very positively: no fever, lower white cell counts, and drainage from the drain in her belly that looks like it's supposed to (I have no idea what it looks like or what it's supposed to look like, but the people who do know and who do look seem happy).

Progress has also been made on several other fronts. She is no longer receiving oxygen, so the annoying apparatus in Sheila's nose is gone. And her catheter has been removed. This is good because it's uncomfortable and a possible source of infection. However, it is also bad in that the only nourishment she's receiving is via IV fluids which lead to the need of using the bathroom a lot—hourly, including throughout the night. So resting is a challenge, but the doctors are pleased that she's moving around and handling the bathroom visits relatively well at this point.

I see additional signs of progress because her personality is becoming more evident. Today, she was a bit fussy. The hospital gown wasn't tied correctly, a medication was irritating her stomach, and, my favorite complaint—"the doctor showed up at 3:00 a.m. and interrupted the Meryl Streep movie I was watching. But at least that's better than when three of them show up when I'm sleeping. I awake and find them just standing there—reminds me of the soloists from "The Mikado." You opera fans might get the analogy. It escapes me completely and I am not planning to look it up. Figuring out how to spell embouchure was bad enough.

Several of you have inquired about whether Sheila needs anything, because you'd like to send her something. I honestly cannot think of anything. She's already received a magnet, stuffed animal, flowers, bookmark, and several other things I can't remember now. Her room is private (thank goodness) but very small and it contains a mountain of equipment. I know she just loves hearing from you and reading notes about what you're doing. So my best suggestion is to keep the cards and prayers coming.

Oh, here's another Sheila classic from yesterday when we were doing the mail. Sheila received a card from her Ohio University friend Gerry, who had included a photo of several OU people taken during a recent reunion of the group. Sheila studied that photo for a few moments and then said, "Well, don't we look like a bunch of used-up sorority girls." So send photos at your own risk!

Even though she is better, the progress is slow. She's still not eating pending more progress with digestive processes getting back to normal (imagine how much fun she's having reporting to all who ask, and many do, whether she's passing gas!). But she is moving around better and usually takes a walk several times a day with her IV pole and a personal care aid in tow. She continues to request no visitors outside of the family. She is too busy during the day tending to all of the things required of her to manage her recovery, and then she tries to rest in between. I appreciate that everyone has been respecting that request.

No big news on the home front. The animals and I are managing just fine, other than that the dog has become preoccupied by a U-Haul truck that appeared yesterday in the neighbor's driveway across the street. She hates that thing and barks at it constantly; I have no idea what to do with a dog who's upset with a U-Haul truck! And Ernie is no help at all—he mostly runs for cover when Hildey gets wound up. I usually manage to distract her for a while, pull the shades, and turn the TV volume up. All of this reminds me why I prefer cats; I've never known a cat to disrupt an entire household over a U-Haul truck!

That's the report for the moment. I hope you all have a great week. Thank you again for your support in prayer and mail for Sheila.

I continued to be scared, despite what the nurses said. It seemed like such good news when they decided it was time for Sheila to eat. She was pleased and perked up quite a bit. But this did not last long. Monday evening was terrible. I walked into her room expecting her to report great progress after she ate. But she was sleeping, mostly unresponsive, and indifferent to my presence, including the mail. She roused herself long enough to tell me that she threw up after she ate and they weren't going to allow her to eat again for a while. I couldn't understand this because the doctors and nurses all said that progress would be uneven, but they would stick with it.

I just sat beside her bed for a while and watched her sleep. It was an effective escape for her, I could understand. She was working so hard to recover, doing what was asked, mostly without complaint. The staff all loved her. They regularly told me that. Even in the midst of significant illness, my beloved friend was extending herself to others.

I wasn't sure what to do. Sheila clearly did not care whether I was there or not. I didn't want to leave her. So I went to the nurses' station for information and was again assured that her condition was the same and that they would continue working with her to get her digestive processes working again.

The following day was more of the same. Sheila continued to be withdrawn and unlike herself, even though she did make an effort to look at her cards. She reported more vomiting when she tried to eat. I tried to have conversation about the dog and even that didn't interest her much. It was no wonder she was dragging. She had been in the hospital for twenty-nine days and there was little end in sight.

I knew I was going to have to be creative with the e-mail crowd, maintaining this balance of painting a realistic picture without getting people alarmed. Sheila continued to tell me that she didn't want her friends to know about the cancer and she wanted my messages to be "hopeful."

1-30-08

I'm a bit pressed for time this evening but thought you would want to know that Sheila has, unfortunately, had several pretty rough days since I last wrote. Things were progressing relatively well until Monday when the doctors decided she should try to eat (broth). That has not gone well. She did not keep it down and has felt fairly sick ever since. Today, the doctors did an extensive day-long test that involved taking pictures of her digestive system every hour (after they injected some dye). No word on results yet.

When I visited earlier this evening, she was absolutely exhausted and feeling discouraged. So your continued prayer and mail support is needed.

2-1-08

Well, the results of the day-long test (conducted earlier this past week after Sheila's poor response to her first eating attempt) are in and things are not good. There is another blockage. This one is "different" from the first that was removed surgically. I'm not sure of the difference. Sheila did not get that part when the doctors visited with her earlier today so she had little detail to relay to me. But she does know that there is another blockage.

The doctors have told her that more surgery is not an option as she is too weak for that. Apparently the nature of this blockage is such that it may resolve itself, and it seems that a blockage like this is not uncommon after an extensive abdominal procedure like Sheila had. So now we wait. There is no medicine that can be given. Her small intestine just has not resumed working since her operation, so without the normal movements in that area, another blockage resulted, as I understand things.

Sheila tells me that the doctors are monitoring all kinds of things as they continue to prepare treatment plans for her—vital signs, urine output, and so on. And she is receiving excellent nursing care. She especially enjoys the nursing students who are there regularly getting practice under the watchful eye of their instructor.

She's working very hard at her recovery and is doing absolutely everything asked of her. She is very disappointed about this new development, however, and her overall condition is very weak despite the IV nutrition that continues to be administered. I know that she appreciates the mail very much and that your prayers are quite important to her. Thank you for your continued support in these ways.

The home front has been relatively uneventful. The U-Haul truck left, thank goodness, so the dog is not obsessing over that any more. We're developing a new routine that we would prefer to abandon when Sheila comes home. I did find myself thinking about the nature of friendship while I was scooping dog poop earlier today. And I think of it every time I find your cards and notes in the mailbox. Wonderful stuff!

I will continue to keep you updated.

It did occur to me that the dog's pen in the yard had not been tended to for the past month. Sheila usually scooped the poop and put new straw down in the outdoor pen area. So I went for a bale of straw on Saturday morning and set out to scoop the poop, a much more pleasant job in the dead of winter, I tentatively concluded.

I really did think about the nature of friendship as I was doing that little chore. I was completely committed to keeping things running at home so Sheila could focus on her recovery. I thought about how much we all missed her at home and how much we loved her. I hoped that what I was doing was right and honorable for our friendship. But it was hard to know for sure. Trying to stay humble about it seemed appropriate. I did decide that, if I ever had tendencies toward over-confidence in my contributions as a friend, a return visit to the dog pen to scoop poop would be a good move.

2-3-08

Sheila had a great day yesterday and a not so great one today. That seems to be the way this is going—up and down rather than several consecutive days of positive progress. Yesterday, she wanted to sit up and talk with me—and was able to do so for nearly two hours. She looked and sounded stronger. Today, she is tired and listless.

I don't understand the treatment plan at the moment. Yesterday, the doctors "clipped" one of the draining tubes to allow all fluids to pass through the digestive system. They wanted to see how that would go for 24 hours. (I thought the plan was to wait to see if the blockage resolved itself). This arrangement went okay yesterday. Today, Sheila ate crackers and Sprite (ordered by the doctor) and they did not stay down. It amazes me that she is not more discouraged. But the doctors do not seem discouraged and Sheila tells me that one of the doctors indicated that they've worked with people longer than this is going on for her. I guess I'm the one who is impatient! So we soldier on.

I know that your cards and prayers are very meaningful. Sheila's most recent comment when I arrived with yet another bundle of cards, "People are being so faithful." So thank you again for your efforts to provide support for her.

On the home front, I took the dog for a walk yesterday and it was eventful. She was actually moving along better than usual (after very carefully selecting several precise spots to do her business and taking her sweet time to do it). We were in Fryer Park across from our house and had just rounded the bend in one of the parking lots when I looked up to see a VERY large dog racing toward us. Hildey was on full alert immediately and I locked the extending leash so she couldn't go far without dragging me along, which I fully envisioned her doing. As this beast raced toward us, I heard a woman's urgent voice (from behind the dog, of course) yelling "Stop, [insert something indecipherable in here]." I could swear that the dog's name was "Killer," but I'm not sure about that. I hung on to Hildey, Killer continued making a beeline toward us, and the woman's shape began to appear over the small hill in the distance.

It was clear to me that the woman was not going to catch her dog before it met Hildey and me. Tomorrow's headlines in the paper flashed through my mind, "Woman and Dog Mauled in Fryer Park." Hildey, by now, did not seem to think this situation was at all threatening. She was dancing in anticipation of great fun. (So much for the watch dog instinct. She must know I'm a cat person, despite my efforts to hide it these days.) The woman loped over the hill and began a full sprint across the parking lot, yelling the indecipherable name all the while, as the beast charged right for us. All I could do was hold my breath and hang on to Hildey. To my absolute shock, the beast came to a screeching halt as she reached Hildey (chicken me allowed her to be between the beast and me) and they engaged in what the trailing woman would later tell me was a "doggie greeting." Egad. As the two dogs sniffed each other, the breathless woman arrived, apologizing profusely and declaring "He's big but he's friendly" all at the same time. And "Don't worry about those noises he's making They sound like growls, but they're not." Right. After some additional pleasantries, I suggested that she go one way and I another, and we parted ways. The dog was a Malamute, just so you dog lovers out there don't think I'm exaggerating about his size. All of this just reminds me to stick with cats.

Anyway, I hope I'm not writing too frequently. I'm trying to keep you updated with enough frequency to be informative. Sheila is holding her own and the animals and I are trying to keep the home fires burning in the meantime. Thanks again for your support.

2-5-08

Well, I'm very happy to report that Sheila has had two pretty good days in a row. She's been taking liquids and keeping them down. Today, she even graduated to receiving a tray delivery at each meal time. She had been suffering from "tray envy" during some of her short walks in the hallways at mealtime when all the other patients received a tray and she never did. The tray contents are not much to brag about. Yesterday was tea and juice, with Jell-O added later. Today the selection was similar with Ensure added. She's really working hard to make herself eat. After the long ordeal of either becoming sick or not eating to begin with, it's an effort for her to make herself eat. But she's doing it.

Other good news of the day is that she took a shower! Sponge baths were the only option prior to today. Sheila said it felt really good. Her only complaint is that hospitals do not provide shampoo. So one of the personal care aids who was assisting her and listened to her wish for shampoo, excused herself from the shower area, was gone a while, and came back with shampoo. Sheila is convinced that she went to a gift shop in the hospital and bought some with money from her own pocket. Isn't it just like Sheila to be the kind of patient who inspires one of the staff members to want to do such a thing? And I received a list of hair care products that have to be delivered in there from her home stash, a delivery I'm happy to make because of the progress it reflects!

The doctors are also now beginning to plan for Sheila's transition home. They're talking to her about continuing to eat, taking short walks and daily showers, so she builds enough strength to come home. Even if she comes home, they will want the IV nutrition treatments to continue, so arrangements for that will have to be made. Discussions are in the early stages, but it is motivating to Sheila to know that, if her progress continues, she can get out of there. She is still very weak and tires easily. Hopefully, she will feel better as her nutrition improves and healing from the surgery continues. The infection is well under control now, but the plan is to monitor that very closely even after she's released from the hospital.

So many of you write notes to me and I appreciate it. I do hope you continue to understand that I am unable to respond to you personally, but I do read your notes and appreciate your correspondence. And, as I suggested before, if you wish to forward these updates to others who would want to know how Sheila is doing, it will help me if you do that. Your cards and prayers are very sustaining for Sheila. Thank you so much for your faithfulness. She continues to request no visitors outside of the family.

All's been quiet on the home front for the past few days, thank goodness. I located the Frosty Paws in the grocery store (finally, after too many attempts during prior visits and my pride preventing me from asking someone where to find ice cream for dogs!), so I have a bribery option available if the mutt really makes me nuts, although I think I've learned that it doesn't take much to distract a dog. Reassuring thought if we run out of the frozen treats.

Sheila was funny talking about her shower experience. "It's way down at the end of the hall past the nurses' station and into the wing where they do the bariatric surgeries. They have a huge room down there for a shower. I guess it has to be large in that wing." I had to laugh. She also observed. "Isn't it something? Those people are in here having surgery to make them eat less. I'm in here trying to get my system to enable me to eat at all."

I couldn't believe they were talking about sending her home. She was weak, unable to really eat, and would need significant care, from my perspective. I was so glad for the progress, but highly anxious about how we would manage. I am not a nurse and had no interest or aptitude for medical things, although the past four years of living with a cancer patient had enhanced my confidence a bit. My mixed feelings were keeping me awake at night. I had to figure out a way to talk to someone who knew what was going on.

2-10-08

Well, as usual, we have mixed news, but the trends are positive. After my positive report in the middle of last week, Sheila had more digestive problems. She was unable to keep food down after a day of pretty good eating. So that was very discouraging and physically draining. She was very subdued for several days and did not seem to come around until later in the day on Friday. It was very hard for her to make herself eat again after such a disappointment just several days prior. She told me at one point "I'm tired of being sick and tired." I don't blame her a bit. She's been a trooper through all of this, but she was really dragging for a few days late last week.

Yesterday, she was a bit better so several determined nurses decided that she was going to get up and go for another shower, despite Sheila's protests that it was too much effort. And I was being the determined (gently, I thought) friend who was going to make sure she ate lunch (if you can call watery potato soup, cranberry juice, and chocolate pudding lunch). So I persuaded her to take several bites of each lunch item (only later was I referred to as "Nurse Ratchet") and I left when the nurses came to haul her out of bed to begin the quest for a shower. All of these activities were ordered by the doctor, lest you think we're a bunch of mavericks in there.

I'm not sure what did it, probably not Nurse Ratchet's approach, but today she was better again. She had breakfast (I didn't ask what that included), we took a short walk and she ate lunch again, this time ice cream, grape juice, and another soup ("dreadful," according to the patient, who also felt well enough to complain that "these people have absolutely no presentation of this food"). Right. Even I can recognize that a hospital tray with "institutional" containers on it is no "presentation."

Other progress late in the week was removal of a drainage tube related to treating her infection, which seems to be well under control. And she had a CAT scan on Friday morning. She hates those, and she's had at least five since she's been in there, because they move her "down to the basement" by way of people referred to as "transport" whose hospital bed driving technique apparently resembles that of a NASCAR driver. Sheila complains of being "bumped around" and getting into elevators that "really should have ramps so you don't feel like your insides are going to fall out when they jam you in there." But the results were good. It seems like the secondary blockage is resolving itself, as hoped. Sheila told me today that the doctor called to tell her that she will have another CAT scan tomorrow (A nurse suggested that she tell "transport" to go slower, that there's no reason they have to hurry. But I doubt that, even if they do, she'll find the experience to be satisfactory). Apparently, the Friday scan was partial and the one tomorrow will be complete. So let's hope for good news as those results are reviewed. And let's hope the patient survives the trip.

Another sign that Sheila was feeling better today occurred when I first arrived. It's been bitter cold here today and I came into her room all bundled up. She was sleeping and I touched her hand with my gloved hand to awaken her. She immediately said, "Oh it's so cold. The poor dog. She must be frozen." You dog lovers out there can just imagine all of the retorts that went unspoken from my cat-loving Nurse Ratchet lips.

On the home front, I can report that the dog is NOT frozen, the cat and I keep each other company quite nicely, and I'm keeping the bird feeders full, per instructions from the patient. The dog walk yesterday was uneventful with no wayward Malamutes anywhere in sight. And I am very grateful to have a stack of cards to take in to the patient each day, thanks to the faithful efforts of all of you. I don't know what words to write to tell you how much it helps to know that good people are supporting us through prayers and mail. Thank you.

I kept expecting a day to come when there would not be a card in the box for Sheila. She had been in the hospital for forty-five days and I had never gone in there without at least two cards in my hand. I thought about setting one aside each day so I wouldn't have to go empty-handed one day, but decided against that. She should receive the greetings from her friends as they came. For as long as I'd known her, she had been a faithful correspondent to people in all kinds of circumstance.

When I barely knew who she was, she sent me a lovely note after I spoke in church. Since I've lived with her, I've observed her efforts to write to kids at church camp, friends in the hospital, and aging relatives. She faithfully sent birthday cards, sympathy cards, and thank you notes galore. She was very good at expressing warm creative thoughts very concisely. People looked forward to receiving her greetings.

She even developed a "grief letter" after Allan died. When she knew someone whose spouse had died, she waited a certain period of time and then sent the letter. She kept a core copy on the computer and edited it for each circumstance. The responses from people were overwhelmingly full of gratitude. "It's time to send the grief letter to so-and-so," she would say. And they would follow up with calls or visits to talk with her, the intended outcome.

Now, it was all coming back to her. Not just because she sent cards, but because of her ability to touch people and to extend herself to them, offering her best kindnesses. The faithfulness of her friends sustained me, too, just by seeing their cards in our mailbox.

2-16-08

I hardly know how to describe this week. It has been full of the ups and downs that seem to characterize this saga for Sheila. Early in the week she was doing quite well with clear liquids and then graduating to puddings and cream soups. On Tuesday evening they brought her a little tray of chicken, mashed potatoes, and green beans and she ate small quantities of all. When I left that day, things were looking very encouraging.

When I arrived on Wednesday, Sheila told me that she had not kept that food down and the doctors told her not to eat anything all day. Needless to say, she was discouraged and so was everyone else (That means me and the nurses. I'm not sure what the doctors are thinking these days. I haven't been there lately when a doctor's been there.) She also received no food all day Thursday. So I was quite surprised when I arrived yesterday and Sheila relayed information that the doctors were again talking about sending her home!

This prompted a bit of a mad scramble to collect some of her things. She's been in there so long that she's accumulated multiple books, trinkets, and toiletries that she immediately wanted me to gather up in preparation for the big move. And we had arrangements to think about here at home if she was really going to come home. The medical people are recommending a hospital bed on the first floor of the house for a while, so we made some adjustment in preparation last evening. Her children have been terrific with visits and other support functions (like moving furniture) for us through all of this.

When she does get out of there, she will continue to need nourishment via the feeding tube, which will mean regular visits by a home health care person. And who knows what else will be part of her discharge orders. So everything was looking pretty good for a transition to home, despite the fact that Sheila is not eating. The tube feeding is apparently the plan for now until her poor battered digestive system heals a bit more.

I talked to Sheila by phone this morning and she did not have a good night. She felt sick despite not eating and was speculating that she may not be released any time soon after all. But she has not seen a doctor yet today and the timeline and details of her possible transition home remain murky at best. She did ask me to let you all know that when she does arrive home, she will continue to request your support via cards and prayers, but will not be up to phone calls or visits for some time. I will keep you informed as events unfold.

All is well on the home front, I think. I'm about to go out for a walk with the dog. It's a beautiful sunny day here and, if I understand dog language, Hildey is requesting an outing. Dogs are so obvious.

Thank you again for your support. I hope you all have a great weekend.

As the Friday developments unfolded, Sheila morphed into her "take charge" mode. Even though I was doubtful about her really being sent home, if she had energy to work on something, I was going to go along with her. She insisted that some of the things in the hospital room had to go home immediately. Not being prepared to receive such orders, it really was a mad scramble to find something suitable to put things in (my briefcase was quickly overloaded) for transport.

And it was a challenge to do the sorting. Some things had considerable sentimental appeal. "Oh, I want to keep that. Mary enclosed it in her card. It makes me think of her every time I look at it." Some things were quickly discarded. "Whatever would I want with these terrible hospital socks?" And some things just had to wait.

We talked quietly for a while about how to rearrange the house to accommodate her hospital bed and decided that the dining room would be the place to set her up. At this point, she announced that she was going to call her son Allan to "help you."

"Sheila, I don't need help. Don't bother Allan. I will take care of rearranging things."

Privately, I doubted that Allan would have time to get involved. He had not been able to visit the hospital much due to work and home demands. And I didn't want to have to adhere to his timeline.

But Sheila was insistent. "He has to get involved in this and do his part. It will be good for him."

There was no point in arguing with her so I at least got her to agree that the best thing to do was to present Allan with two options for meeting me at the house to do the work, later Friday evening or Saturday morning. His choice. If none of those times worked, I would handle it. I was sure I could find help if I needed it. So many church friends consistently offered to do anything, and they always emphasized "anything" that we needed. As it turned out, Allan was available to meet me later that evening.

As all of this planning suggested, Sheila was quite certain that she was coming home. I was trying very hard to be positive about that possibility without revealing my secret anxiety regarding our ability to manage her being there. At this point, I wasn't taking one day at a time. I was taking two hours at a time

Allan and I really had a relatively simple job to do. Our table was a drop-leaf with boards in it. We took the boards out, dropped the leaves, and pushed the table right in front of the window. The small china cabinet was pushed into the corner and the area rug was rolled up and moved to the basement. We carried the chairs to the basement, too, and pushed the small desk into a corner.

I was trying to create an arrangement in my head that would allow Sheila to look out the window if she was in bed. She loved our yard and the beauty of nature. We had three beautiful serviceberry trees right outside the dining room window that would be blooming in the spring. I suggested the arrangement to Allan, who readily agreed. And we thought that our rearranging resulted in plenty of room for the hospital bed.

After Allan left, I stood back and looked the situation over and realized that we needed some additional things. I started my mental list, trying very hard to anticipate Sheila's needs while envisioning how to make our dining room an appealing place to recover.

The next morning, I was off to Kmart. I don't ordinarily frequent Kmart, but it seemed like the perfect option for things that would be put to temporary use in our house. I bought a large tension rod and curtain to hang up in the doorway from the dining room into the front hallway. People coming into the house should not immediately see Sheila in her bed and she should have privacy whenever she wanted it. I had measured before I left and was pleased to find things that would work. The curtain was blue, Sheila's favorite color.

I also bought two no-skid throw rugs, one for each side of the bed. I thought the hardwood would be cold and uncomfortable to step onto, so was pleased to find two blue throw rugs that would work. I bought a Rubbermaid set of stacking drawers in which I envisioned we could keep things like washcloths and other supplies that might be needed to tend to Sheila's needs. All in all, it was a successful trip. I was proud to have thought of everything. After unloading my loot, I went to the hospital to report on the progress at the house and to see if the patient had any more information on plans for her release.

Weekends in hospitals have a different pulse to them, as I learned over the seven weeks I had been visiting. Many of the week-end staff are temporary employees and doctors are hard to find. Sheila had a rough night on Friday, so we agreed to not get our hopes up about her discharge. I still felt major discomfort at the thought of being responsible for her care once she was released. I decided to take the immature approach and pretend it wasn't happening. I was just trying to be positive and encouraging with Sheila.

Fortunately, Connie and Claire stopped by, so I left. I thought it was a good opportunity for her to talk to someone other than me and I didn't want to impose on their time with her. I went back that evening to check in with her and to get another load of her stuff. She was tired, but feeling better at the thought of going home.

On Monday, things got hectic. I came out of a morning meeting to find a message from Sheila in my voice mail saying to call her as ASAP. She sounded fine, so I wasn't scared. I probably should have been. I called her immediately and she told me they were planning to send her home later in the day, but we had some things to organize. Could I please talk to the social worker about her release plan?

"Of course," I told Sheila, trying to sound completely confident and comfortable with this whole idea. I called the number Sheila gave me, with my pulse rate increasing as I dialed. Today? She's coming home today? Despite the dining room preparations, I didn't feel ready. But I couldn't resist. It meant everything to Sheila to come home.

"Suck it up, Nancy," I kept telling myself. The social worker was very thorough with her questions about the layout of the house: Yes, there is a half bath on the first floor. Yes, I live with her and will be the primary care-giver. Yes, there is a working telephone in the house. Yes, we have a safe place for a hospital bed. No, there are no weapons or illegal substances in the house. No, there are no other people, just a cat and a dog.

I realized that I had just claimed the role of primary care-giver, but it was evident to me from recent experiences that Connie and Mark would not be able to take this on because of their work and family responsibilities. And despite my serious reservations about my ability to do it, I wanted to claim the job. I was the person closest to Sheila and I knew her better than anybody. We had promised each other that we would stick together and help each other. It was time for me to step up. So I claimed the primary care-giver role without giving anybody else the option to have it. My uneasiness about it, on a scale of 1-10 with 10 being on the verge of panic, was 9.5.

The social worker told me she would order the hospital bed and other equipment to be delivered to the house later in the day. "Can you be there this afternoon to meet them?"

"Not until after 4:00 p.m.," I replied. I had some pressing business issues that required my attention that day. I knew I had to maintain the balance between work responsibilities and home responsibilities. What I was discovering was that work was turning out to be quite therapeutic. It required my full attention while in the office, so I could not be distracted by what was going on in the hospital until I got to the hospital.

Fortunately, the social worker could arrange the deliveries for after 4:00 p.m.. I went racing from the office, past the hospital, to home to meet the hospital bed delivery person, trying to stay focused on the task at hand rather than my own increasing anxiety at the thought of Sheila sleeping in the dining room that night.

I had to get home and receive these deliveries and get back to the hospital quickly so Sheila would not have to wait one minute for me. I wanted to be there so when the discharge procedures were completed, I could get her out of there. The social worker told me that the doctor was doing this because they were hopeful that a move home would improve Sheila's morale. He was worried about her getting depressed. No wonder. She had been in the hospital for forty-eight days. The doctor also thought that perhaps moving around at home would help her digestive process be restored. "Good plan," I kept telling myself.

As I drove home, a panic thought hit me. A hospital bed was being delivered into which Sheila would slide her weary body in a few hours, and I had no sheets to put on the bed. All the beds on our house were double or queen size. I was pretty sure I had no sheets with which to make the bed! I couldn't stop to buy them. I might miss the delivery guy. It would be unthinkable if I had to tell Sheila that she couldn't come home because I missed the bed delivery. I was running late as it was and had to find a solution.

I went racing into the house, flung open the door of our linen closet upstairs and began a frantic search through the shelves for single bed sheets. As I had expected, there were none to be found. I raced back down the steps, grabbed the phone book, and dialed the number of a neighbor two houses down who had repeatedly told me she would "do anything" to help Sheila. No answer.

Church friends lived one street over. Surely they would be home and would be in possession of single bed sheets. I dialed quickly. No answer. Aggie wasn't home either. The good thing about this immediate crisis is that I didn't have time to think about how in the world I would care for Sheila once she got home.

Not able to think of anyone else to call, I tried Lisa and David. Lisa answered the phone, to my immediate relief. A live person to help me solve this problem! "Lisa, Sheila is coming home this evening. A person will be delivering a hospital bed sometime very soon, so I cannot leave. I don't have any single bed sheets to make the bed up. Do you have single sheets at your house that we can borrow until I can get to the store to buy some?"

"No, all the beds in our house are double or queen."

My heart sank. I could feel my frustration level approach an unhealthy state as I asked myself, "How could I not have thought of this? What am I going to do? I want her bed at home to be warm and comfortable and I don't even have properly-fitting sheets to put on it!"

As I was thrashing myself for my oversight and trying to figure out whom to call next, Lisa continued, "Don't worry about it, Nancy. I'll find sheets for you and we will bring them over. I'll keep calling people until I find some."

She took my problem for herself. I let out a sigh of relief and thanked her profusely. I knew she would deliver. And I knew David would help her. These two had taken their Sunday School lessons to heart and were living with generosity and unselfishness. It was another perfect response from my friends. I took time to remind myself to be like them when I grow up.

After the bed had been delivered, David and Lisa showed up with the sheets and helped me make the bed. I was eating a cup of yogurt and talking to them when the IV pole installer arrived. Once everyone had left I headed back to the hospital. I drove Sheila's car because it would provide a more comfortable ride than mine. I wanted Sheila's trip home to be as smooth as possible. I was half-laughing at myself thinking that I didn't want to be accused of being in the same category as the hospital transport crowd, which never met her standards at all.

When I arrived at Sheila's room I found Mark with his mother and, after about an hour of waiting during which I had time to think again about the challenge before me, the nurse came in with discharge instructions. There were two prescriptions for Sheila to take and a reminder that the Home Health Care nurse would be arriving later that night to teach the caregivers how to use the tube to feed Sheila. She had to have food supplements because her own system still didn't work correctly. Mark offered to get the prescriptions filled while I drove Sheila home.

I could not help but think, "Isn't there a better way to discharge people from the hospital than to send them home needing to have prescriptions filled immediately?" Seriously. It also was snowing heavily and blowing and here I was driving an unfamiliar car with an unwell person with me. That drive was the most tense fifteen-mile trip I think I've ever driven. It must have taken forty minutes to get home, as the roads were slick and visibility poor. Amidst all of this, I was trying to exude calm confidence. My mind was busy anticipating a long list of events for the evening, all of which made me tense and left my stomach in knots, though not primarily because of the road conditions.

When we got to the house, Sheila commented about how good it was to see the place. That made me smile inside. I backed the car into her side of the garage and stopped before the car was completely in. This allowed her side of the car to be closest to the door into the house and for the car door to avoid a support pole in the middle of the garage. I felt bad about the cold air coming into the garage, but thought that direct passage to the house was the priority for the moment.

Before I could remind her to take it slow and easy, Sheila opened her car door, swiveled her hips sideways, stood up, and took off toward the door into the house. I raced around the back of the car and arrived behind her just as she opened the door and put one foot up on the step into our laundry room. She was awkwardly hanging on to the door knob behind her, trying to pull the door closed, a move she had done thousands of times over the years. However, this time, her legs were not strong enough to navigate that one step and she crumpled to the ground, half in the laundry room and half in the garage.

The snow was swirling into the garage, Ernie was standing there alert to the possibilities, and the dog was barking hysterically in her little room behind us. There wasn't room for me to kneel beside her, so I stepped over her, turned around, and knelt on the laundry room floor to look at her face. "Sheila, are you hurt?"

"No! But I don't think I can get up. I'm not hurt. I'm sorry to be such a bother."

I said silently to myself, "Nice, Nancy. You do all this work to prepare a place of comfort for her to be in the dining room and give not one thought to how you're going to get your patient into the house," as I considered our next move, while reassuring Sheila that we could handle this.

"Just rest for a minute," I said. "I'll be right back," as I decided to get a chair from our kitchen in the hope that if Sheila could hang on to it, this might help somehow. Sheila then expressed her own concerns, "Ernie's going to get out and Mark won't be here to help for a while. What are we going to do?"

While Sheila was calm, at that moment we could not see a way out of our predicament. I kept asking her if she was hurt and she kept insisting that she was fine. "It's just that my legs are weak." How I was wishing that the social worker had asked about entry into the house, too.

I put the chair right in front of Sheila and asked if she thought she could use it to help herself on her knees into the laundry room. Any competent medical person watching this probably would have been apoplectic. I wanted to call the squad to come and help her get up but she rejected that notion out of hand. "I can do it if I rest for a minute," she assured me.

I then got behind her in the garage and lifted her hips while she used the chair for leverage and we got her into the house. But that only got her to the floor of the laundry room. I was completely paranoid that we were hurting her, but Sheila kept insisting that she was fine. The dog settled down a bit and Ernie wandered away after he determined that nothing going on would result in food for him.

Sheila rested again while I considered whether we could get her from the floor to the chair. I repositioned the chair so she could grab both the end of the washing machine and the edge of the chair. After a brief waiting period for her to rest, Sheila announced that she was ready to try to get into the chair. I got behind her again and grabbed her hips.

"On the count of three, Sheila. One, two, three!" I lifted her as high as I could and she pulled with her arms and pushed with one foot and we launched her into the chair. I knelt in front of her and looked right into her eyes to assess her state of mind, if nothing else. She was breathing heavily from the exertion and I was over the top with anxiety.

"Nobody would believe this, so let's not tell them." she said with a slight twinkle in her eye and a weak smile. "Thank you for being here. I always know I can count on you." If I hadn't been so traumatized myself, I might have cried in response to her high complement.

Fortunately Sheila snapped me back to the task at hand. "Help me into a chair in the family room. We want to look like everything is normal when Mark and the others get here," she said.

On the way through the kitchen, she paused in the doorway into the dining room to review the set-up, but didn't spend much time in that assessment. It was getting late and we still had a ways to go. She settled contentedly into a chair in the family room while I went back into the garage to unload some stuff, get the car the whole way in and the door closed.

Not long thereafter, Mark came with the prescriptions and Connie arrived. She had been invited by her mother to come for the briefing that the Home Health Care nurse would be doing about how to care for her. We never did tell anyone about her trip into the house that evening.

Orders for Sheila were to try to eat anything liquid that she wanted. The main source of her nutrition would be through a tube that had been inserted during her surgery. It exited from her left side and was attached to a bag that handled drainage. But it was also useful for feeding. How to use it properly was the primary lesson we were to receive from the nurse. The arrangements were that the nurse would call when she was on her way.

We sat and waited, making small talk while Sheila occasionally dozed in her chair. Connie helped her get into a fresh night dress, robe, and slippers, all of which proved to be an exhausting effort after such a day as she already had.

I was highly anxious and impatient as time dragged on. Sheila was finally home and I wanted to have some semblance of normality now that the both of us were in our home for the first time in months. And, mainly, I wanted her to get some rest. I knew that she was tired. I was tired and extremely stressed from the racing around and anticipation of the care-giving that was facing me, not to mention Sheila's visit to the laundry room floor. The days of Sheila pushing a call button and having a highly capable person show up were over. Now, it was going to be up to me. And I was not at all certain that I could do the job for her.

I had no idea that Home Health Care nurses were expected to run around in the snow at such late hours. But Mary was completely unperturbed by the weather or the hour, as far as I could tell. Her instructions were clear and she assured us that they were only a phone call away. I felt a little bit better then. Just a little bit. As she went out the door, she said; "You'll be fine. You have common sense."

After Mark and Connie left, I helped Sheila to the bed, imploring her to call me when she needed to use the bedside commode. She said she would, but I could tell that she had other plans. She could not persuade me to sleep in my bed upstairs. I was determined to sleep on the couch in the family room, so I could hear her if she needed anything.

My night was filled with anxiety and I was particularly afraid Sheila would fall getting out of the bed in unfamiliar territory. I wanted her to feel secure, that someone was nearby who would respond if she needed anything. My mind was full of fears and insecurities about my ability to care for her properly. The arrangement was that Mark was coming back in the morning. It was his day off and he would stay with his mother while I went to the office. In the morning Sheila was sleeping when I went upstairs for a shower after I had tidied up the family room. I was pleased that the night was uneventful for her and I will admit that I wasn't worth much at the office that day.

2-20-08

Sheila came home from the hospital on Monday evening (in a snowstorm, of course, so it took us forever, in keeping with the overall struggle she's had). She had a very big day on Monday being excited to come home and doing several things needed for her release. So she was really tired by the time we got here about 8:00 p.m., but she has been doing better each day.

Her children and I are learning about how to care for her, since we're operating a home hospital room, trying to do everything the hospital staff was doing while she was there. It's been an interesting experience to be part of the great machine of medical care. Monday was a day of conversation with the social worker, nutritionist, home care coordinator, medical equipment truck dispatcher, and several others I can't even remember.

Ben, the hospital bed fellow, arrived first and took great care to get the bed set up properly. Next to arrive was the medical equipment fellow, Andre, who put the IV pole together, primed the feeding pump, and provided several other supplies. After that was the Home Health Care Nurse, Mary, who arrived at 11:00 p.m. to begin teaching us the procedures needed to provide home care for Sheila. The nurses provide guidance and oversight, but the caregivers do most of the work. By the time we were finished with all of the instruction, it was almost 1:00 a.m. Mary was a real trooper and I was doing my best to not disclose my Nurse Ratchet tendencies.

Sheila is very glad to be home, but still feels very weak, as expected. We're working on getting the volume of her tube feeding just right. The volume has been too high in the first few days and it made her sick, so we're consulting with the nurses and making adjustments. Her children and I are taking turns being here with her during the day to handle administration of medications and additions to the feeding tube. We have a very compliant patient who seems to be getting better each day. Let's hope that pattern continues.

Sheila continues to request no visitors and we trust you understand. She still loves the mail and asks me to let everyone know that she feels your prayers, so please continue those if possible. We've made positive progress but have a very long way to go.

Ernie has determined that the hospital bed is an ideal location for him to bathe elaborately and then sleep contentedly. Good news is that he stays in the basement during the night, so he has not attempted to do this at the same time that Sheila is in the bed. She gets up and sits in a recliner during the day so she "doesn't feel like a sick person." This is good.

I decided last week that the poor dog needed a bath and haircut, so had made an appointment for her to be beautified yesterday. Then I realized that I had to get her there. I obviously had no idea what I was doing because I had never transported a dog anywhere for any reason. I soon learned that an excitable dog riding in a car calls for some combination of self-defense, childcare skills, and just plain commitment to get the job done. I was not convinced we'd survive the trip! At least the semi-crazy people at the grooming place were glad to see her—and even sent her home with bows in her hair. I thought they were kidding when they said they would "make her pretty for Sheila." This dog thing is really a revelation.

Thank you again for your support.

Despite my anxieties about caring for her, Sheila's presence at least felt like our household had regained its natural order. Unfortunately, however, the home care regimen was not going well. Sheila was feeling sick most of the time and was clearly not absorbing the liquid food. I could see it draining back out into the discharge bag not long after it was administered to her. It was so hard to take her back to that hospital. I knew she didn't want to go, but wanted to feel better. I packed her up and took her in. It was profoundly difficult to leave her in that hospital and drive home alone. I had to keep telling myself that the doctors would figure something out that would feel like positive progress. The house felt especially lonely that night.

2-21-08

Well, you might have expected the path to be less than smooth, given the way this journey has gone for Sheila. The disappointing news is that we had to take her back to the hospital this evening. As I indicated in the previous note, we were struggling to get her tube feeding regulated so it, plus the medications administered through it, would not make her nauseated. We were not able to strike the right balance as indicated by an all too regular need to remove some of the nutrition in order to prevent Sheila from being sick.

After three days of this, the doctor determined that she needed to go back to the hospital to resume feeding via the IV because of a concern that she was becoming dehydrated. This surgeon is highly invested in Sheila's recovery and has a bedside manner that is reassuring and compassionate. He had given his pager number to Sheila when she left the hospital and wanted her to call him personally today to report on how she was doing. It was during this conversation that he decided to readmit her.

Sheila is disappointed but told me; "This is where I need to be right now. I know that." She went right back to the floor where she had been treated previously (she was very glad about that) and most of the staff greeted her with disappointment about the fact that she had to return, but they all started requesting assignment to her because they know she is pleasant under unpleasant circumstances and shows interest in every one of them. Sheila told me that the doctor said she'd be there "for three or four days." I'm not sure if that's wishful thinking or if that is the case.

Your continued support via prayers and mail would really be appreciated. I know it means a lot to Sheila to hear from you and we're both impressed by the fact that you're so consistently providing what she needs despite the length of this journey.

As for the balance of this disappointing day, the dog and I are going to watch the hockey game, Ernie's resting comfortably in the hospital bed that he has now claimed for himself since the patient left, and we're all going to hope we have enough bread and milk in the house to survive the little snowstorm that's underway.

Goodnight for now.

2-24-08

Sheila has had several fairly good days in the hospital. Her lead doctor told her after he reviewed her test results on the first day after she went back in there that her nutritional status was "not as bad as I thought it would be." That was reassuring news to me, one of the caretakers who had been responsible to administer her tube feeding properly.

I can tell that she feels better because she has been awake each time I've arrived for my visits, unlike the weeks prior when she was almost always sleeping. Her conversations indicate that she is more involved in events around her as evidenced by our visit today. As I hit the doorway to her room about noon, she saw me coming and announced, "This has been a very frustrating morning." As I inquired about why that was so, she explained, "The tubes on this IV machine had to be replaced because they were driving me crazy."

In the instant I had to think about that statement, I was having a very hard time imagining how plastic tubes from an IV machine (exactly like the kind she's been dealing with for weeks and weeks) were causing so much frustration for a veteran hospital patient like Sheila. Only a true musician will sympathize as the explanation unfolds.

"They were making dissonant sounds, a B and a C, I think. And then when the nurse call signal in the hallway was added to it, it became completely intolerable because that is a B, too." Oh, my.

This is what we refer to in local circles as a Margie moment because Margie is a fellow musician from church who always nods her head understandingly when Sheila comes up with these things, while I stand there being completely incredulous trying to gauge whether Sheila is kidding (usually, she is not). And she wasn't today.

Apparently, a nurse had come to the rescue and changed the tubes, so harmony was being restored just about the time I got there. I must say that I'm pretty sure that, had I been there earlier, I would not have noticed "dissonant" sounds coming from IV tubes!

When I told Sheila that I thought this story would be good fodder for the e-mail update, she nodded her head thoughtfully while contemplating my suggestion and then said; "You do know how to spell dissonant, don't you?" I promptly accused her of being under the influence of a nausea drug that was making her mean. At that moment, someone across the hall had a wicked coughing fit and Sheila said, "Hairball." I rest my case.

Speaking of nausea, she had some trouble with that later today, but doesn't seem discouraged by it, mostly because the doctors and nurses don't get rattled, I think. Her doctors have told her again that she will be there "for a few days," so her morale is pretty good because of the prospect of coming home again in the not too distant future. I surely hope it works out that way. She did not see the doctor in charge this weekend, but I imagine she will see him tomorrow, so perhaps the plans will be clearer then.

The home front is doing fine. Ernie is annoyed with me at the moment because I removed the bedding from the hospital bed and washed it so it's all fresh when Sheila comes home again. Remember that Ernie had claimed that bed for himself after Sheila left. I did provide him with an old blanket that I thought was perfectly fine, but he's boycotted the bed since, just to let me know that he prefers the nice stuff that was on there for Sheila. Too bad.

We did have enough bread and milk to survive the weekend snow. And we have the unendingly generous support of friends and family that helps us survive this medical and emotional challenge. Sheila said to me yesterday when I went in with yet another handful of cards, "I can't believe how faithful people are in sending cards." When I asked her if there was anything other than the IV tube difficulty that she wanted me to tell you she said, "Tell them all that I feel their prayers."

Thank you all for your continued support.

I came home today with a folder full of instructions on the proper care of a PICC (peripherally inserted central catheter) line. That's what they decided Sheila needed. It would be the new means by which she would receive nourishment. This called for another lesson from another nurse on how to properly handle such a procedure at home.

We knew that a one week's supply of the feeding liquid would be delivered and that it had to be refrigerated. Assorted other supplies also were being delivered to the house. I had to meet people there to receive the deliveries. It was a massive amount of material, including pre-filled saline tubes, back-up batteries for the pump that will push the fluids through the line, sterile gauze wipes, and too many other things to mention.

My anxiety level was way up again. I was not really looking forward to another evening training session with another visiting nurse. Mark and Connie were also coming. I was also quite worried about the untreated cancer. The longer this went, the longer treatment for the cancer was delayed. I understood that they wanted Sheila to be stronger. But sooner or later, we had to get to

Dr. Cohn. I kept asking Sheila if I could mention the cancer to her friends and she kept asking me not to do that. It was weighing on me to handle her care and to keep this secret.

Eight more days in the hospital. I don't know anyone who has been a hospital patient for fifty-six days. No wonder they wanted to get her home. I was holding on to what the doctor said when I was discouraged, "We think we can get her through this."

Before her discharge this time, I resolved to have a better arrangement for getting her into the house. I wasn't going to have a repeat of the laundry room collapse. So the night before, after everybody was fed and the mailbox emptied, I tried to think of what to do. I remembered some extra bricks that we had stacked out in the yard. I thought they would be about the right height to make a very low step that Sheila could handle, even with weak legs. I bundled myself up and ventured out into the yard with a flashlight, making sure the dog was in the house so she wasn't out there being hysterical at a hooded creature thrashing around in the yard with a flashlight.

I located the pile of bricks under the snow and was beginning to feel smug about the brilliance of my plan. But I soon discovered that the bricks were frozen together.

Ok, back into the garage for a hammer. I held the flashlight under my chin and slammed the hammer into the pile of bricks, dislodging several from the top of the pile. I took another whack and several more tumbled down. I made several trips to get them into the garage where I spread newspaper and allowed them to dry out for a short while. Slipperiness would not do for this project. When I got the bricks inside I also realized that they would not be thick enough to provide relief from the tall step.

The thought of venturing back out into the cold windy night with the hammer was none too appealing, so I tried to think of something else that would work. Surely there was something in our garage that would do the trick. I began to search and, sure enough, I found the cans of Coca-Cola we had stored out there in their dispenser-like containers of twelve. I was never so glad to see a box of Cokes in my life. I put one at the foot of the door on the garage floor and it was a perfect height. From the top of the box into the laundry room was a 3-4 inch step.

I placed several Coke boxes sideways to make a nice small platform, and then got to work on the bricks. I put them on the garage floor, too. Their heights created a smaller platform that led to the Coke boxes. I put a towel over the bricks to stabilize them and tested our new steps into the house. It seemed like I had a satisfactory solution. I would discover later that it worked perfectly for Sheila's return home.

2-28-08

Well, we have several news items to report today. Sheila came home again as of late this afternoon. Arrangements have been made for a different kind of feeding that is expected to prevent the dehydration problems that developed using the previous method. The home health care nurse is arriving shortly to teach us how to properly administer this new method.

I was with Sheila yesterday when her chief doctor came in to review her situation with her. He advised that there is a new blockage that explains her lack of progress with eating. Apparently, they've been watching a troublesome area during several recent scans and he has now concluded that there is a blockage there. He is baffled about why there seemed to be a blockage present—then there wasn't and now there is again. He would like to think that this one will resolve itself, but is not optimistic that it will. Sheila requests specific prayers on this point, that this new blockage will resolve itself.

In the event that does not happen, she must have additional surgery. She is home now because they still want to strengthen her physically and psychologically. The doctor said; "We'd like to get you out of this hospital environment for several weeks and help you feel stronger before we do anything else. So that's what we're working on now.

The doctor will be monitoring Sheila's condition via phone each week. He wants to talk with her every Monday. He does not want her to go through the effort to make a trip to his office, sit and wait, etc. It is inspiring for me to see his commitment to her and his personal investment in her treatment. He told her that, despite the need to treat this new blockage, he's very optimistic that they can treat her condition and see her through this. So again we pray for this to be a very positive outcome.

Your continued notes and cards and prayers are so helpful that I don›t know how to express how much it means to know that so many people care about our situation and take time to be involved in these ways. This has already been a long haul and more effort is required. Sheila and I talk about the blessings of this situation and there are many. One significant one is the blessing of each of you. Thank you.

Time to go learn how to be a nurse at home!

I was glad for the presence of the nurses as I learned to meet Sheila's needs. They were very patient with a medical novice like me. Someone came each day in the early evening to watch me do the hook-up of the IV pump that had to run for sixteen hours. They explained that most people like to hook it up on the evening and sleep with it running so they can be untethered from it the following morning.

After consultation with Sheila, we agreed on this approach as well. Connie and Mark and I took turns being there in the morning for the unhooking. I handled all the hook-ups with them providing back-up. This was a major responsibility and I tried not to think too much about it for fear of becoming overwhelmed. Each time I finished the hook up, Sheila said, "Thank you." She was always gracious.

I was pushing for physical therapy so Sheila could get stronger physically. She was very lukewarm about the idea but I thought it would be good for her and told the Home Health Care nurse that. She agreed and ordered it. As a result, we had multiple callers and visitors in and out of the house to get these services set up. I just hoped that all of it would lead to positive progress. We needed to feel positive progress.

Sheila gave me permission today to tell her friends about the evidence of cancer. But she was again emphatic about my being positive and not assuming a "prophet of doom" approach to the e-mail updates. She had been feeling better and I believed we should disclose the information so her friends could get used to the idea. Hopefully, we were not too far away from a consultation with Dr. Cohn. I really wanted to hear his assessment of Sheila's condition.

3-2-08

I am pleased to tell you that Sheila has had three fairly good days here at home under the care of her children and me. She's so happy to be home and continues to work hard on her recovery. The new feeding and hydration approach seems to be working, as evidenced by her getting a little stronger each day rather than weaker as had happened before when she was home.

We are working on establishing a routine and need more time to get comfortable with everything. Sheila requests your continued support via mail and prayer, but asks that she receive no visitors or phone calls for a while longer. She will be receiving visits from a physical therapist, nurse, and personal care aid (maybe more, but that's what I know for sure at this point). The frequency of these visits is unclear at this time. Most of the interactions so far have been for the purpose of getting us started with the IV administration. I did it without supervision this evening for the first time. It's totally intimidating to have so much responsibility in a field that is so unfamiliar to me, but since doing it is necessary, I'm tackling it with the attitude that it's part of the role that I need to play in all of this.

Sheila receives her IV "feeding" and hydration fluids starting in the early evening. These IVs run for 16 hours. Thus, she can be disconnected for 8 hours each day. During the disconnected time, we've been taking walks around the house (she announced today after I had prompted her to walk "I don't know why they're sending a physical therapist with you around here") and improvising her bathing routine.

Her daughter Connie and I tried assisting with bathing and hair washing yesterday. Sheila was a real trooper and it is a wonder she did not drown. But she felt better and Connie and I felt like we did something positive for her. I must say that I think this bath and hair washing consumed a record number of towels. We had water everywhere, but the patient came out of it clean and happy. I'm hoping the personal care expert will offer some tips that will make us more effective next time.

Sheila's medical plan is to get stronger so she can withstand further treatment that she needs. If her new blockage does not resolve itself, that will require surgery. The doctor has also advised that there was some evidence during the surgery that her cancer may again be present. So part of the treatment plan is to get her well enough to proceed to her oncologist for a review of her situation. Her primary doctor (Dr. Chambers) was emphatic that he thinks they can get her through this, so we continue to work on not getting ahead of ourselves.

Tomorrow will be Sheila's first phone call to Dr. Chambers, who we hope will be pleased to hear about the quality of the care she is receiving and her overall progress. Each time someone comes and goes from the house during this teaching process for IV administration, I envision them going to their cars and completing a form to indicate their confidence in the caregiver. I'm thinking the question is something like "On a scale of 1-10, how confident are you that the caregiver has a clue?" I hate to think what they're reporting.

On the home front, the dog and I survived two walks this weekend. Yesterday, we were in the park moving along nicely (finally, after extended bouts of excessive sniffing and shifting inches before squatting) when up over the far hill (opposite hill from our Malamute encounter) came the heads of three people. I did not consider this to be a problem at all—until it became clear that they had two leashes, which I assumed contained two dogs. When I was able to see the end of the leash that contained a dog and not a person, I could see that these dogs were relatively small, so I was feeling somewhat like the Malamute owner must have upon seeing us—no problem! Hildey by now was extremely interested in interacting with these two, one of which was wearing a silly, really bad doggie sweater—purple with ugly designs on it. The killer was that the young man in the group was strolling around with no jacket—only a T-shirt—apparently trying to impress the young women. The dog was dressed more warmly that the adult.

Hildey, as expected, charged ahead, I hung on, and the little dogs retreated behind the young women holding the leashes. Those little things were absolutely not interested in doing a "doggie greeting." It must have been the sweater. My dog intimidated their dogs—and mine didn't even bark! I was almost proud. Nobody said a word. The little chicken dogs ran in the opposite direction and I dragged a disappointed Hildey away.

This evening, I was sitting on the couch and Hildey jumped up beside me and wanted attention. Sheila says that the dog now thinks I'm the "leader of the pack." She must be kidding. I'm not interested in being the leader of a dog pack. Just my luck to be identified by Sheila's dog as her new best buddy, even now that Sheila's home. I think she's only trying for special favors because I'm her only source of exercise and food (I meant the dog, not Sheila, but, now that I think of it, this applies to both of them!). I'm not a soft touch, however.

We're doing OK here. Ernie the cat sleeps at the foot of Sheila's bed each morning (after I get him out of the basement where he spends the night) and she likes his company. She generally stays in the bed until the IV feeding is completed and then spends the day in her favorite chair that provides an excellent view of the outdoors and the TV. Being here is doing wonders for her morale, even with me as chief nurse and self-appointed physical therapist.

I hope all is well with you and yours. Thank you again for your support and encouragement.

Connie brought the baby monitor that I requested so I started sleeping upstairs again. It was true that I would rest better, but I was paranoid about Sheila's needing something and my not hearing her. Sheila was making her new room quite comfortable, rearranging things on the table near the window. I changed the family photos for her so she had new things to look at for a while. I thought we were settling down a bit. Mark was there twice a week and Connie took a day. I had the other two days and week-ends. I was hoping for that consultation with Dr. Cohn soon.

3-6-08

Our patient has had several fairly good days, other than the morning drama today, which I will tell you about shortly. But the most important news is of Sheila's improving health and the continuing progress that we are all making in establishing a daily routine.

Sheila is gaining strength each day. She now walks to the bathroom on her own when not tethered to her IVs. She's reading the daily paper, watching TV shows of interest to her, and making occasional phone calls to family members. She rests relatively well, although has to get up every few hours to use the bedside commode because the IV is running all night long. Not a great arrangement, but at least she can be disconnected from it during the day (the IV, not the commode. She's never connected to the commode.).

Several new professionals have been added to her Home Health Care staff. We met Jennifer, the physical therapist, this week. For my money, she's perfect. She's a no-nonsense type with a very warm personality who will not allow the Gallipolis girl (who did everything possible to escape PE class) to weasel out of doing recommended exercises to improve her balance and strength. So far, the exercises are very basic. I can hardly wait for things to become more demanding. I may have to invite Nurse Ratchet back for a return engagement to provide support for Jennifer.

We also met "Scotty" this week. She's the personal care aide who's otherwise known as Mrs. Scott. She's been in the business of serving people for many years and it's obvious that she loves her job. I held my breath, though, when the therapist alerted us to Scotty by saying, "Oh, you'll love her. She sings while she works." Oh no. An amateur singer, crooning to a music major with a highly sensitive musical ear. I envisioned a possible calamity and immediately began formulating a plan to psych Sheila into loving Scotty no matter the quality of her singing. I wasted my time. Apparently, Scotty indeed "has a lovely voice" and the two have hit it off. And Scotty is completely unintimidated by the fact that our first floor contains only a half bath. Best of all, her husband is from Steelton, Pennsylvania, my dad's home town. Only Sheila would have collected that information after one visit with a personal care aide.

The drama of the day began when I heard Sheila calling me about 5:00 a.m. When I arrived at her bedside, she said, "My tube must be leaking; I feel something wet here." Upon investigation, it became clear to me that nothing was leaking. The tube had completely pulled out of her belly! I'm no medical person, but even I could tell that this was not good and would require consultation with the Home Health Care team. I plastered a calm look on my face and tried to keep an even tone in my voice when I told Sheila I thought we had to make a call to get some advice. She agreed.

This home care team is very responsive and there was a nurse on the phone with me within minutes asking several pertinent questions. "What kind of a tube is it?" (I don't know - it's clear). "OK, what does it do? Do you feed her through this tube?" (No; we give medicine and it drains unneeded fluids from her digestive system). "How much of it is still inside her belly?" (None, as far as I can tell; how would I know what's still in there?). At this point, she announced; "I think I'll page the doctor and call you back." (Good idea!)

Sure enough, she called back in a very short time and said the doctor wanted me to try to "see if you can put the tube back in." (Are you kidding?) "Try to lubricate it with something (What do you suggest?) and push it back in as far as you can." (Expletive!) Sheila looked highly skeptical when I announced that this was the plan. But I was determined to try. The nurse had explained that getting it back in would be good so the opening in Sheila's stomach would not "close up." So I told Sheila to take a deep breath (saw that on TV once) and I pushed, got the thing part way in, told the nurse, who then said, "Now call the squad to take her to the ER so they can reinsert it fully and confirm that it's OK via x-ray." Right. Now things were looking up, from my perspective.

When I told Sheila that she needed to go to the ER to have her tube reinserted properly, she was not so positive. She tried to persuade me to take her so she would not have to endure that "bumpy ride" (I pointed out that she'd get treatment faster if she arrived via squad, so she gave in), then immediately announced that she needed to change her gown. OK. Got that done. Let's dial 911 now. Got that done. Squad's on the way.

As I was beginning to relax about handing her off to people who know what they're doing, Sheila said, "What about my hair!" Of course. A person has to have great hair at 5:30 a.m. for a ride to the ER in the emergency squad vehicle.

Got the hair combed. So my patient was now reclined on her bed looking resplendent with her hair combed, brand new freshly laundered pastel bed gown flowing around her with matching slippers on her feet. I suddenly realized that I, on the other hand, was standing there in my bare feet in a faded flannel 10-year-old night shirt, holding part of the cast-off G-tube, with my hair looking decidedly like I was a loser in a Pebbles Flintstone look-alike contest. "Sheila, these squad guys are going to think I'm the sick one!"

Sure enough, when I opened the door, a very earnest-looking young man took one look and said, with appropriate professional concern in his voice, "Morning, ma'am. How are you feeling?" I promptly redirected him toward the person in the hospital bed and went to get the list of Sheila's medications.

Things turned out fine. The ER was not busy, Sheila received attention promptly, her tube was properly reinserted, and she was back home (thanks to her son Mark) within several hours. She's tired this evening, but not really any worse for the wear. And neither am I.

So that's the news of the day. Again, I thank you for your consistent support via mail and prayers. We truly feel the network of concerned friends and family who are with us in this. We do regularly say thank you prayers for all of you.

Of course, I had a major meeting at the office on the morning of the ER visit. I was not thinking about it when the drama was unfolding. But once the squad left with Sheila and I had assured her that I would be following close by, after taking a shower and making myself presentable, I realized what day it was and that it would be a good day for me to be in the office, if I could possibly make it.

Mark was scheduled to come to the house to be with his mother that day anyway, so I felt like I could contact him to go to the ER to pick her up and get her home. I waited until a humane hour to call him and breathed a sigh of relief when he answered the phone. I quickly explained the situation, assured him that his mother's condition was not at all urgent, and asked him to meet me at the ER.

As I drove to the hospital thinking about Sheila and about my meeting preparations, I was starting to feel overwhelmed. I knew I was physically and mentally tired. But then I thought about Sheila lying in the ER after an ambulance ride, and I realized that I was not the one with the challenges. And she was so brave and so uncomplaining. She never lamented her condition, instead saying that her mother always said, "Something's going to get you." She would then say, "I don't know if this is going to get me, but I'm going to do everything I can to get well." She was compliant with me and the doctors and the other care-givers who tended to her. I resolved not to feel sorry for myself. But I did think it was time for me to take some time away so I could remain strong for whatever would be coming.

3-12-08

Well, things are finally boring in our world! There is really not too much to report about what's been happening for the past few days. Sheila continues to get stronger and the doctor wants to see her on Monday, presumably to assess her progress first hand and discuss next steps in her treatment.

She is working very hard at her recovery. She does exercises each day to strengthen her legs and hands. The physical therapist was very pleased when she visited this week, so that was encouraging. We did our own version of physical therapy on Monday when Sheila made her way to the piano for the first time in four months. She was able to sit and play for a little bit and it was a wonderful moment that made us both cry. She had been concerned that she would lose her musical ability and was very tentative about trying. She needed not to have worried. The skill was still there. She was not able to play for longer than a few minutes, but it was a very positive moment.

Sheila's children and I are taking turns being here in our home with her during the day to handle the "unhooking" from the IV feeding and administering a few basic medications. The nights have calmed down. Sheila still has to get up every few hours, but is able to do that, so I'm getting much more sleep than I was early on.

Next week I will be on vacation from my job and will travel to Pennsylvania to visit my family and friends there. I'm looking forward to it and appreciate the support being provided by Sheila's family that makes the trip possible. Her brother is planning to visit from Alabama and that will be good for both of them.

Sheila continues to appreciate the mail from all of you and the prayers that provide incredible spiritual strength to her. Thank you for your continued commitment to these things. Thanks also to many of you who write to me. I feel your support, too. And it means a lot. I will write again as things unfold here.

I received one of the great compliments of my life during one of these days. One of the kids had been here and left when I got home. Sheila spoke about how much she appreciated what they were doing and then said, "But I feel the most confident when you're here."

I was pleased when she persuaded me to do the morning unhooking and then go to work. She was insisting that she didn't feel uncomfortable being alone for a while and in fact, liked it. She kept a phone nearby and assured me that she was not out of her mind and would know who to call if she needed help. I was a bit skeptical that she was just worried about imposing on me, but she persisted in her argument that it was senseless for me to work from home twice a week all day.

I agreed to a one-day trial. She was fine when I got home and expressed a wish that her children would follow the same routine. She never did persuade them. I took the occasion to talk with my boss about this schedule, now that it seemed like we were on to something that might be predictable. I offered to use vacation time or leave time to cover my morning absences for a few hours twice a week. That idea was quickly rejected. "You do what you need to do. You work plenty of hours. I don't need to know which days you're doing what. Just put it on your electronic calendar so I know where to reach you if I need to." Another great gift when I needed it resulting in one less thing to worry about.

I began talking to Sheila about my going to Pennsylvania for a few days. I needed a break and wanted to see my friends and family there. We talked about who would provide coverage during my absence. Mark's work schedule was such that he could not be available in the evening to hook up the IV and Connie said she felt overwhelmed at the thought of doing that. So we arranged for the nurses to cover for a few days and Sheila called her brother in Alabama.

To his credit, Steve readily agreed to come to be with his sister. But I was not totally relaxed about the arrangement because I knew there was longstanding underlying tension between Sheila and her brother, built up over a lifetime of sibling interactions between two strong personalities.

I was especially anticipating the visit to Dr. Chambers since he was in charge of her care at the moment. I wanted to hear what we had to do that would equip us to move along to Dr. Cohn.

3-17-08

Well, the doctor visit today was satisfactorily positive. Dr. Chambers was very happy to see Sheila and was very pleased with her overall condition. I asked him if she looked better or worse than he expected, and he said she looked better. I think the man has a future in politics. Sheila, of course, told him that she'll look even better next time he sees her because she'll put her make up on before she comes. Always the sorority girl.

He remains concerned about the new blockage and says that he is "perplexed" about its development because on one post-operative scan, her small intestine was "running smoothly" and on a subsequent one, there was a new blockage. He's not sure what's happening in there now. You will recall that he said sometimes these things resolve themselves, but he was not optimistic that would happen in Sheila's case. But we've all been praying hard that it would happen that way and that no additional surgery would be necessary. Now he wants to do another scan. And he wants to see her again in two weeks. He's also in consultation with her oncologist because of concern that her cancer is again present. There is no appointment with the oncologist until she's over this intestinal problem, as I understand the plan.

Sheila was dressed today for the first time since she's been home. That was an adventure, especially with the tubes and attachments she has. But she's learning to work around them and I like to tell her that she's "free to move about the cabin" when I unhook her from the IVs in the morning.

I'm leaving for my visit in Pennsylvania tomorrow morning. Sheila's brother Steve arrived this morning and has been observing the various care activities that she needs. I think they'll do fine and I'm looking forward to the changes of scenery for a few days.

Thank you again for your continued support in prayer and mail. Sheila is getting stronger, thanks in some measure to her determination to do it and the knowledge that so many people care about her.

Helping Sheila get dressed was fun for us, in some ways. She was feeling good about being well enough to go out, even if it was to a medical appointment. We had survived the adjustment to life with a PICC line. That required another trip to Kmart, where I bought some colorful (blue!) gowns that snapped down the front, for easy in and out. But the PICC line went into Sheila's clavicle area, so putting her arm in a sleeve was a challenge. I recruited a friend to cut the sleeves in the gown I bought and modify them with snaps, so Sheila could get in and out of them comfortably.

Regular clothing didn't seem like it would be an issue because the IV line wasn't running. It wasn't, but we had to be careful with jeans. We learned that Sheila's jeans fit in a way that made them impossible to wear because of interference with her drainage tube.

We laughed for a while at the thought of her going to the doctor pantless and then recovered ourselves in time to think about a pair of sweatpants I had. They had a drawstring, so could easily accommodate whatever was inside them. Sheila and her tube with discharge bag fit easily. And I kept telling her that I didn't recognize her in regular clothes. She laughed. That was music to my ears.

3-24-08

I know it's been a while since I've written to update you on how things are going in our world. I thoroughly enjoyed my visit with friends and family in Pennsylvania last week. Sheila and her brother did well while I was away. When I came into the house on Saturday evening, the first thing Steve said was, "Look, she's still alive!" And she looked great to me. Last week, Sheila continued to undertake more daily activities for herself. In fact, on Sunday morning when I came down the steps,

I found her already relocated to her recliner in the family room with IV pole at her side and Easter music on the TV. That reflects her growing confidence in her physical condition and her ability to handle things on her own, I think.

We also took a big step yesterday when Sheila went up the steps and took a shower for the first time. It's quite a process to prepare for the shower because it involves covering her IV line and G-tube with plastic to prevent water from touching them. I was chopping up garbage bags and unrolling tape while Sheila described the process used by the nurses in the hospital to perform this function. Then, Ernie the cat arrived to offer supervisory support while the dog barked hysterically at the neighbor's grandchildren. Sheila was terrific and had plenty of energy to stand in the shower, do her hair after the shower, get dressed, and come back down the steps. Then she promptly fell asleep in her chair for a short while. It was so encouraging.

The scan that the doctor ordered last week is scheduled for Wednesday. We have to travel back to the hospital for that. I don't know when the doctor will receive results, so we will keep you posted on any news that comes from this. I know that Sheila is eager to get on with the next step in her treatment and is getting tired of being tethered to the IV for 16 hours each day.

The biggest nonmedical news of the household this week is Sheila's announcement that the grandfather clock is "out of tune." I did not know that clocks went out of tune, but this apparently is a problem of some distraction because I've heard it mentioned several times in recent days. "That clock sounds abominable." I usually say something not helpful like "I don't know who to call to tune a grandfather clock" in response, while envisioning a poor soul on the other end of a phone listening to me explain that the clock keeps perfect time, but requires service because it's out of tune. If anyone local knows who tunes clocks, let me know!

So for this week, we're back to the schedule we've developed with Sheila's children and me taking turns being here to unhook her IV in the morning and assist with some of the personal care activities that are still too much for her. It's a great collaborative effort and we're all encouraged by Sheila's progress, even though we recognize that she still has a long way to go.

Your cards and prayers continue to be a great blessing and I know that Sheila looks forward to the mail each day. Thank you for your faithfulness in this ministry to her. We do appreciate you very much.

3-29-08

We have had a pretty good week. Sheila continues to do more things, although slowly and with long periods of rest in between. She's in a routine now of going upstairs, getting "taped up," and taking a shower each morning. That's good exercise and it makes her feel ready to take on the day, I think. She's also reading the newspaper each morning and occasionally watching movies or other TV shows. One nice day this week, she even walked to our mailbox and back to retrieve the mail. Too bad we don't consistently have nice days so she could make that a regular routine.

There was a bit of trauma this week. We went to the hospital on Wednesday for the scan the doctor ordered. Easy for him to order, but not so easy for us and the technicians to deliver. Before we even left the house, Sheila expressed concern that "they're going to make me drink that awful stuff and I'll throw up." She knows this routine all too well from having had multiple scans before and during her hospital stays. I tried to put a positive spin on it by telling her that I thought the doctor said they would put the dye in her tube and she wouldn›t have to drink it. I really did think I heard that. Maybe it was wishful thinking. But she felt somewhat better (maybe) as we started up the highway.

I dropped Sheila off at the hospital door and went to park the car. When I came back to pick her up for the walk to the testing center, I found her in a highly animated conversation with one of the personal care aids who had been a favorite during her hospital stay. This woman went on and on about how good Sheila looked and how nice it was to see her "vertical." I never thought about that—that most hospital caregivers do see their patients either horizontal or sitting. As we moved on, Sheila reminded me of this woman's life story, which she had learned and remembered, of course. She was feeling very good about this reunion and we were off to a fine start.

After registering at the testing center, it did not take long for things to deteriorate. We waited for just a few moments until a friendly-looking technician emerged through the door with a full glass of stuff in her hand and another container of something ominous-looking in the other hand. "Mrs. Zinn?" she inquired loudly to the room full of patients and their drivers. She approached as Sheila waved her hand. "OK, time to start drinking your contrast solution. Are you allergic to anything?" Expecting full cooperation and a negative answer, she stopped dead in her tracks, swishing the dreaded liquid over the edge of the cup and on to her shoes when Sheila said, "Yes, iodine. And if I drink that, I'll throw up." I loved it. But I recovered from my moment of glee quickly enough to suggest that perhaps they could apply the contrast solution via Sheila's G-tube, as the doctor has suggested. The young lady then had to simultaneously try to clean her shoes, consider what I had said, contemplate the impact of the iodine allergy, and assess whether Sheila was being difficult or if there really was an issue here.

So she plopped the glass of stuff (what was left of it) and the other container on the table beside me and said, "Don't let her drink that," (Are you kidding?) and went off to consult with someone about these unexpected developments. Before she left she asked two questions, "Have you ever had one of these scans before?" I actually laughed this time as Sheila very patiently explained that she had been a patient in the very same hospital for many weeks and had multiple scans, but she was sure that if she drank that stuff she'd throw up. The technician then ask Sheila, "Where does your tube go?" By this time I was impatient. (LOOK IT UP. SHE WAS HERE FOREVER AND YOUR STAFF PUT IT IN! YOU HAVE VOLUMES OF MEDICAL RECORDS FOR HER.) But I kept quiet while Sheila said she wasn't sure where it went.

The technician came back in 10 minutes or so and said that the radiologist said that it would be OK to use the tube to get the contrast into Sheila's belly, but since they had not planned to do it that way, we had to wait until their lunch hour was over (about 15 minutes) when someone would be available to do it. (I will never understand why they would not have known that a person who has not ingested anything by mouth for weeks and weeks should have her contrast dye inserted via tube and therefore should have planned accordingly). And then she'd have to wait about an hour to begin the test. I then asked, "OK, may I come back there and wait with her until you're ready to do the test?" The technician snapped, "Oh no—that would violate patient privacy. I'm sorry." (What? And one of you coming into the waiting room full of people and announcing your patients' names very loudly does not violate privacy!). I was getting grouchy at this point. So, as previously agreed upon with Sheila, I left when she went to get her contrast via tube, by now almost an hour after we arrived.

When I came back to the waiting room about an hour later as planned, Sheila was not to be seen. I waited for almost 45 minutes and finally saw the second technician who had come to pick Sheila up to get things started and asked him if Sheila's scan was finished. "No, it hasn't even started. She threw up all the contrast dye. It turns out her tube goes into her stomach. So they're back there trying to figure out what to do." Terrific. But it wasn't too much longer until Sheila and a third person emerged from behind the closed door (the one through which nobody but patients can pass due to privacy but the very same one the staff uses to come out and announce all names. (Can you tell that whole thing make me nuts??!!) Sheila is looking quite weary, but steady on her feet. They explained that they thought they finally got enough stuff into her system to complete the test.

Sheila very politely thanked the person with her and we moved toward the door. As we walked out I didn't say much until she absolutely cracked me up by saying, "Sure enough, they insisted on giving me three full glasses of that stuff and I gave it right back to them."

We go to the doctor on Monday. He wanted this test to see what's going on in there and to provide him with information to recommend next steps in her treatment. Once we know more, I will update you.

Thanks again for all your support. We are very much sustained by your careful attention.

Even though we made good progress in terms of Sheila's improved strength, her overall condition was still a concern. We'd been working to get her digestive system to work and it wasn't happening. I was so glad that she was strong enough to occasionally go for a ride in the car with Mark or take short walks because it seemed like an enhancement in the quality of her life. Her morale was amazingly good and my anxiety settled down as practice made me more confident. But we were both getting impatient about going back to see Dr. Cohn.

I had been trying to keep things light with the email correspondents, in keeping with Sheila's wishes. She regularly reminded me to keep the notes positive and to downplay the cancer. I was trying to strike the right balance, because I thought these faithful people deserved truthful messages from me. Thus, I included the entertainment of the household goings-on, which people seemed to enjoy.

3-31-08

The trip to the doctor's office was uneventful, thank goodness, because the test results are worrisome. Dr. Chambers, who has been treating Sheila since the first of January and who has been wonderfully attentive and available, told her that the results from last week indicate that the cause of her current digestive trouble is the formation of a tumor, they think. He explained that he saw some evidence of malignancy during her January surgery but it had not formed into a tumor; it was "granular." But he says that the radiologist believes that the blockage they are seeing on the scan is from a tumor that has now formed.

Dr. Chambers said that he does not think Sheila is a good candidate for surgery at this time because she remains generally weak and her recovery would be terribly long and difficult. He thinks it is a better option to pursue other treatments.

This means that Dr. Chambers is referring Sheila to her oncologist, which Sheila and I are happy about. Not that Dr. Chambers and the people at Mt. Carmel haven't been great. They have been. But this change presents the opportunity for treatment by a doctor with whom Sheila has had a relationship for four years and who has access to one of the finest oncology hospitals in the country at OSU (It pains a Nittany Lion to say that.). Dr. Cohn is terrific and Sheila already has an appointment for next week. He and Dr. Chambers have been consulting by phone on her case and he apparently agrees with this approach.

We're trying hard not to get ahead of ourselves by anticipating treatment options or possible outcomes, although my mind is busy with this constantly. Sheila is occupied with lamenting the things she cannot do for other people until she feels better and worrying that she's "taking too much" from her children and me. I tell her we all owe her and that things have been out of balance with her giving and our taking for a long time.

We had a great weekend here. Sheila went to visit her daughter Connie for a short while and rode around in the car with me while I did a few errands on Saturday afternoon. Then she went to church on Sunday. That was big. Both outings were an effort for her, but made her feel good, I think, and enabled her to see something other than the inside of our house or the hospital. We're trying to make each day better than the previous one.

We ask for your continued prayer and mail support while next steps are decided. Sheila feels your prayers and delights in your cards and letters. I try to keep her loose and laughing while providing care in a manner that causes her no anxiety. Her children and brother are all a source of strength to her as their faithful attention is received.

Thanks to those of you who write to me expressing thanks for the e-mails. I hope you do understand that I am not able to respond to you individually as these group notes are the best I can do. Thanks also to those who provided leads on a person who might tune the clock. No progress on that yet. First things first.

I will update you when there is more news.

Anticipating the oncology consultation made me highly anxious. Sheila was not eating, despite her best efforts. The nutrition in the feeding liquid was making her stronger, but she clearly was not well. It had been months since we learned of a cancer recurrence and I wanted to know what Dr. Cohn recommended. And then again, I didn't.

I was thankful for Sheila's improved energy and ability to do things. I tried to suggest additional things for her to do that would continue to improve her morale. I suggested that she receive visitors, thinking that seeing her friends would boost her morale. She rejected that suggestion saying she just didn't feel up to it.

I encouraged her to write her own e-mail update and she declined to do that. I suggested that she come to church with me for an hour, just to sit and listen to handbell practice. She wasn't comfortable with that idea either. These were stark reminders to me of how much she was unlike herself, how far away she was from her healthy self. It scared me and tested my resolve.

4-7-08

We've had a relatively routine life in our household for the past week. Sheila continues on her IV feeding and is now occasionally drinking clear liquids. The IV runs for 16 hours and the contents are determined by her weekly blood tests. We receive a delivery of the new prescription IV food every Wednesday. She is receiving all needed nourishment through this process, is not hungry, and is maintaining a healthy weight.

I connect her to the IV each evening between 5:00 and 6:00 p.m. and the person who is here the following morning does the "unhooking." I learned this week by accident that Connie and Mark, two of Sheila's children, started referring to me, the handler of the opposite function, as "the hooker." No wonder this label has been under cover.

Sheila is also going up the steps every day for a shower. She has also started doing some computer functions like making cards and occasionally viewing e-mail herself. But this depends on her energy for the day. She is sometimes tired because her nights are not restful. The IVs cause a need to use the bathroom every few hours. So she is up and down a lot at night.

News of today is that Sheila's appointment with her oncologist was this afternoon and he presented her with two options. She can do nothing, allow the cancer to progress, and it will end her life. Or she can choose to receive chemotherapy. He explained that the spread of the cancer suggests that it is more aggressive than was previously evident. He wants to provide her with a good quality of life for as long as possible. He outlined the risks of chemotherapy and stated that, should she choose the treatment option, he would recommend an approach he called "chemo light" that has been even curative (25% of the time) in some patients with conditions similar to Sheila's. But he reminded her that chemo certainly has risks and Sheila is well aware of those, having been through chemotherapy previously.

Sheila is now taking time to consider this decision. She's called her children (Connie heard this first hand because she went along for the doctor visit) and her brother this evening to let them know what the doctor said. If she chooses to receive treatment, it would begin in several weeks. The doctor said there would be benefits to waiting because it would allow her more time to recover from the ordeal of her surgery before the chemotherapy would begin.

I asked Sheila how she wanted me to conclude this e-mail. (She has been aware of the content of almost all of these, except for a few when she was in really rough shape in the hospital.) She said "Tell them that we remain hopeful and trust God for the outcome."

That about says it! Thanks for your prayers and cards. Please keep them coming.

The consultation with the oncologist was quite sobering. Dr. Cohn was his usual effective self. I have so much regard for that man. He handled Sheila perfectly and imparted information with confidence and compassion. He told her that she would have six months to live without chemo treatments. I had to grab the arm of the chair to control my reaction to that one. We'd gone from doctors telling us that they were confident they could bring Sheila through this to hearing that she had six months to live without chemo.

After he explained the chemo option, I asked him; "What is a best case scenario in terms of outcomes from the treatments?" not knowing what to expect given his prior presentment.

"I've known people to have similar conditions who respond well to chemotherapy of this type. I've seen it be curative. We have every reason to think that you will respond well, based on your prior experience," he said, turning to Sheila.

I was hanging on to the word "curative" and watching Sheila's face to try to see what she was thinking. I was surprised when she said she wanted to think about it.

I wanted to jump up and say, "No!! There is no thinking about it. You have to do it. I need you to be alive. I need you here." But I kept quiet, including on the ride home. My mind was racing again. None of this was what I had expected.

Sheila asked me what I thought and I told her that I would support whatever she decided. Her illness was hers alone, I told her, and I was confident that she would make the right decision for herself. It was the thinking side of me that said those words. The emotional side of me wanted to lobby hard for chemo. Telling her that I would support whatever decision she made was a very hard thing to say. But I loved her and respected her too much to say anything else.

4-11-08

I just have time for a quick report this evening but wanted to let you know that Sheila has decided to undergo chemotherapy. Her first treatment will be April 24. There is quite a bit of pre-work that must be done, including drugs, tests, etc. Those activities begin several days prior to the treatment, so we will be busy. And she most likely will not feel too well for several days after the treatment.

I would say that Sheila's had a pretty good week. She's working on getting stronger and has taken short walks outside when the weather cooperated. She's also doing a few small things around the house (light laundry, emptying the dishwasher, etc.). She continues to appreciate your mail and prayers very much. You have been so faithful and it means a lot. Please don't stop now.

Thank you for all your support.

Sheila really was enjoying the fact that she had a bit more energy. The fluids that were feeding her were miraculous. The nurses called Sheila each week and asked her about her weight and several other questions, so they could adjust the formula in the liquid food. I had to laugh one day when Sheila described one of the calls from the nurse and the specific question about her weight.

"How did you tell her what you weighed, Sheila? Did you go upstairs to a scale to weigh yourself?"

"No, I lied", she replied with a great big smile on her face.

"Sheila, she's trying to help you. Why would you lie?"

"Because I felt like it. I've worried about my weight most of my life. I'm not doing it now. They can just keep sending the same formula. It's working fine."

"Have you lied to the nurse all along?"

"Yes, she calls every week and every week I make something up. I do try to remember what I said last week so I don't say something outrageous."

I decided not to fight that battle. She could have some control. She was so patient with everything else that was swirling around her. If she wanted control of her weight, she should have it.

I was so pleased when she decided to undergo the chemotherapy treatments. I would not have felt that way had Dr. Cohn not indicated that treatments could be curative. Sheila had gone through so much. If there could be a recovery from this saga, I wanted it to be. I recognized that Sheila knew what to expect and admired her courage. We didn't talk about it much, other than to agree that we would do the best we could with it.

4-19-08

Sheila hasn't had a very good week, unfortunately. She's having trouble with pain and nausea these past few days and it is really bothersome to her. We had a rough night on Wednesday into Thursday and I finally got on the phone to both doctors' offices and insisted that someone do something.

The trouble started, I think, when Sheila developed a urinary tract infection ("UTI," as the professionals refer to the condition). That required the addition of a new antibiotic to her regimen of medicine which had begun the week before. When it seemed that she wasn't over it, we had called the surgeon's office on Monday and learned that he was out all week, but the doctor covering for him provided an extension of the medicine (after a second call to prompt a response). I think the new medicine was causing the problem.

Sheila's nausea and pain increased as the week went on. By Thursday early morning, I knew we needed help and that nurses couldn't do anything without a doctor. I decided to start with the oncologist's office so Sheila's situation could be reviewed by someone who really knows her. The nurse there was terrific, responding, "She's in pain? That's terrible. There is no reason for that. What are you giving her? How much?" I felt like I was connected to a woman of action, which is precisely what we needed at the moment.

But this wonderful nurse believed that medical protocol, a complete mystery to me, called for me to talk to the surgeon's office. So I called there, described the problem and the young lady suggested that in Dr. Chambers absence, I should take Sheila to the ER. What went through my mind at that instant is not something that I can put in writing to polite people like all of you who are reading this. But I said, "No, I'm not taking her to the ER. Do we have another option?" The woman said she would check with one of the doctors in the office and let me know.

About that time, the oncology nurse, Annabelle (by this point she and I are on a first name basis), called back to see how I made out. When I told her, she responded by telling me that she would get Dr. Cohn's approval for anti-nausea medication and an upgrade to Sheila's pain medicine. Great. And she got it done in a reasonable amount of time! Independent of this action, Sheila and I had already decided the day before that she would quit taking the new antibiotic, so by Friday she was feeling somewhat better.

However, throughout this past week we have had too many occasions when there's been a need for the "barf bucket," a sickly pink-colored plastic hospital-issue device relied on by care givers and sickies everywhere. We have three of them scattered in various locations around the house so we're always ready if a need arises suddenly. And it sometimes does. We've also learned that the device can be multi-functional. Sheila converts one of these barf buckets into her "Ernie helmet" each morning and evening. Ernie is our 16-pound cat who loves to visit with Sheila when she's in her bed and he's not confined to the basement. But he wants to walk on her. So she turns the tub upside down and rests it on her stomach as a deterrent to this persistent cat. It's quite effective.

Ernie also felt called upon to provide supervision this week when one of the nurses was here to change the dressing on Sheila's IV lines. This is a highly specialized process. The nurses must have told me a million times when she first came home, "Don't try to do anything with these. ONLY NURSES can handle this." OK. Got it. I have enough to handle without volunteering to venture into territory that's out of my league. So when they come to tend to this thing, they're very serious. They put masks and gloves on and tell Sheila to turn her head and not breathe on the area. Apparently, Sheila and the nurse of the day were intent on this process one day and neither of them saw Ernie approaching to express interest in the proceedings. I guess he jumped onto Sheila's lap, causing her to scream and the nurse to smack him and fur to fly. I think the image is pretty hysterical. But Ernie's been confined to the garage or basement every time since that incident when the nurses are here!

The household mystery of the week is how three perfectly formed whole robin eggs landed on our brick front porch. How can that be? If they fell from a nest, they would have broken, we think. One theory is that the robin ate too many berries, was tipsy, and laid them right on the bricks! All bird-watchers are welcome to offer a theory.

So we've made positive progress in the past two days. I asked Sheila what she wanted me to say today and she said, "Tell them there are so many positive things. I love looking out at the pretty spring flowers in the yard. The birds provide endless entertainment. And I receive so many nice cards and letters from people. Those cards and letters make me feel best. When people write, it's like having a little visit from the person and I like that. Be sure you're not negative!" How can I be when I'm caring for a person as sick as she is who has this kind of attitude?

This week is the first chemo treatment. A blood test will begin the process. This is used to track progress, as a baseline CA-125 reading is taken before and after the treatment. It is one indication of progress. The treatment is Thursday and Sheila will see the doctor after it is completed. The treatment is in his office and the entire visit will take two to three hours. We do remain hopeful and appreciate your support in prayers and cards.

Thank you for being there for us.

I decided that I wanted to be the person to go with Sheila to her chemo treatment, but didn't want to interfere if she had ideas about one of the kids going along. She hadn't said anything about the plans, so I brought it up and was pleased when she said she preferred that I go, but didn't want to cause problems with my work schedule. I assured her that I could arrange to be out of the office for the day, if I could check in via phone occasionally, which was easy to do.

I had become fiercely protective of her, even when she was in the hands of her doctors. I learned about the importance of a patient advocate during medical procedures throughout the hospital marathon. I was determined to remain vigilant as we began this chemo journey. We were both optimistic that there would finally be a breakthrough and Sheila could continue with a strong recovery.

4-26-08

It's been an interesting week. Since I last wrote, Sheila's been to a place called the I.C.C., had her first chemo treatment, the downstairs toilet leaked, and Hildey and I experienced the return of the Malamute. Let's go in order.

Early in the week, Sheila continued to have significant nausea and pain issues. The little pink tubs were being used all too frequently and her morale was sagging, understandably. (Mine would have been completely in the dumper months ago.) But she quietly (usually) tolerates it all while I get impatient to do something that will help her.

On Monday morning, I called the oncologist's office to speak with Annabelle, my new hero, who listened calmly to my description of our patient's condition and then announced, "She needs to be seen. (Oh, no. I know what that means.) She probably has an intestinal blockage (her hero status slipped a notch at this point - WE KNOW SHE HAS A BLOCKAGE!). You don't want to go to the ER (back to hero). I'll make a reservation in the I.C.C. They will probably want to scan her (visions of Sheila making her "if you make me drink that stuff, I'll throw up" announcement). Do you know what that is and have you been there?" (No and no).

Annabelle explained that the ICC is the Immediate Care Center at the OSU James Cancer Hospital that treats patents referred by their doctors for immediate attention. The doctor's office alerts the staff there that someone is on the way and they provide a general time frame for the patient's arrival. I thought that option sounded terrific. Sheila didn't, so we did not go. Despite my best persuasive efforts, she wanted to wait to see if a few more days of the previous medicine would improve her symptoms. Good thing I don't make my living selling anything.

On Tuesday, Sheila's son Mark was here for the day. After yet another visit with the pink tub, they called the doctor's office again and received a referral to the ICC. Their reviews of that place were stellar. The patient is ushered into a private room, waiting arrangements for friends and family are quite accommodating, and the staff is highly attentive. So while the doctors figured out what to do, Sheila and Mark watched the flat screen TV in the room. But more important than any of that, the medical staff decided not to scan Sheila but changed her medication and sent her home with assurances that this stuff would work. It has! It took a while, but was worth it.

Somewhere in the midst of these proceedings, the toilet began to run continuously. Because our very lives will have to be in danger or the house on the verge of collapse before repair people will darken the door, I decided to fix it myself. Fortunately, a toilet is not a very complicated device. Sheila was skeptical, but agreed that it was our best option. And the noise was bothering her, of course. With her musical ear sensitive to all sounds, this toilet was causing considerable disturbance. At least she didn't analyze what key the noise was in, as has occurred with other household noises. So I dove in and, after several trial and error efforts and a small measure of frustration, the repair was completed.

One beautiful evening this week when Sheila was not engaged with the pink tub, her IV was running fine, Ernie was asleep on the blanket on her bed, and the toilet was quiet, I decided to strap Hildey's harness on her and take her with me for a walk in the park, thinking it would do us both some good and Sheila would be pleased. All was well as we crossed Orders Road and began our trek along the road into the park toward the YMCA and ball fields. I was lost in thought about whatever I was thinking about as we walked along, until Hildey suddenly began to prance and dance excitedly, pulling in the direction of the woods about 30 yards away. She sometimes thinks she sees things and makes moves like this, so I did not completely come out of my meditative state but just tightened my grip on the lease. But it soon became apparent that Hildey was not experiencing a minor distraction.

A great thrashing and crashing noise from the woods began to thunder across the field and I could not believe my eyes when I looked up to see the Malamute (on a leash this time, thank goodness) charging from the wooded path into the trees and underbrush in a wild attempt to come and greet her doggie friend Hildey. The woman on the other end of the leash was hanging on for dear life, narrowly missed being dragged into a tree, while I came out of my trance in time to forcibly restrain Hildey from charging into the woods from the road. The woman finally managed to get her dog to halt his quest while I contended with Hildey, while a guy driving by in a pick-up yelled the classic, "Who's walking who, there?" In a few moments, the humans recovered and made the disappointed dogs move in opposite directions and we went on our way.

Thursday was chemo day. It went well. Sheila's treatments occur in her doctor's office, which offers a calm environment with highly competent and caring staff all around. While they were running late by about 30 minutes, they soon got Sheila situated in a very comfortable chair, used her existing PICC line to hook her up, and her treatment was underway. She felt very good that day (must be all of your prayers), so we decided that we deserved a treat. Big spenders that we are, we went to McDonald's and I ate ice cream and Sheila sipped on an iced coffee as we drove home. It was humbling to be in that chemo treatment room. Sheila and I both commented about how fortunate she is to have access to medical professionals like them. And we were both reminded that, sick as she is, there are patients more ill than Sheila who are persisting to battle their disease, too.

Dr. Cohn stuck his head into the treatment room to see Sheila and asked if her new medication was working. He explained that his resident had come to talk to him (while he was in surgery and Sheila was in the ICC) to decide what medication to give her. He was very pleased that the new regimen was working. And now we know why the treatment was not immediate. The resident had gone to consult with the chief doctor.

Since Thursday, Sheila has been feeling OK. She takes several additional medications specifically for post-chemo purposes and those are going fine. No visits with the pink tub since Tuesday, thank goodness. She's tired and having trouble with bladder control, something that is typical of patients who are immediately post-chemo. She asked me to tell you all that "the treatment went fine and we won't know anything about results for a while."

The next few days will not be comfortable for her. The medical staff is careful to explain that days three and four after chemo are typically when the patient feels the worst, so we have to plow through that before things will get better. Sheila generally is not up to having company or even talking on the phone. And she's not working her e-mail either. She does continue to look forward to the mail delivery each day, so we appreciate your continued attention to her in this way and through your prayers.

I know this is long and I'm still using the distribution list that Sheila prepared months ago. If you'd rather not receive these updates, please let me know and I will remove your e-mail from the list. Thanks again for your support. We truly appreciate it.

We were both feeling pretty good about how things were going. We talked about how we could envision an end to this long haul, thus my offer to the email people to drop out. None of them did, amazingly to me. And it continued to be true that our mailbox contained at least one greeting card for Sheila each day. She cherished those little communications from her friends.

Some people even started sending cards to me, too. I was touched by that thoughtfulness. I'm not sure it would have occurred to me to try to sustain the caregiver. One message written on a card really impacted me: "There is divine and human appreciation for what you are doing." I held on to that thought fiercely. I hoped I deserved it, especially the divine part.

5-3-08

Since I last wrote, we've spent a day in the ER and Sheila has been in the throes of her post-chemo sag. Ernie the cat, Hildey the dog, and I have not been anywhere, which is a good thing.

The ER saga was last Sunday. Sheila got up feeling pretty well and even considered going to church. But after her shower, we discovered that her G-tube was leaking significantly, as it had the night before. We had thought the previous night's problem was a flukey thing related to post-chemo medications and overall fluids flowing through her body. But when it happened again, I knew it had to be tended to. We called the OSU resident physician on call who responded very promptly, agreed that the tube needed attention, and said that the only option was an ER visit. Oh, my.

I tried the argument that Sheila would "be seen" more quickly if we called the squad, but she countered with "but we should not tie up those nice men with this when someone else might need them more and I'm perfectly capable of getting there in the car." I had no worthy comeback for that, so we piled in the car about 10:00 a.m. and took off.

I could relate a lot about our ER visit, but won't bother you with the details of the day. Suffice it to say that Sheila was amazingly cooperative and good humored about the entire thing despite being three days post chemo when she was supposed to be feeling the worst, if the nurses in Dr. Cohn's office are to be believed (and they are). I, on the other hand, was mostly grouchy and impatient with the outrageously slow pace of things in the ER. We were there for almost four hours before anyone even resembling a doctor looked at Sheila. We finally got home about 4:15 p.m., with a new G-tube and an exhausted patient.

Sheila has otherwise responded well to her treatment until about Wednesday when she really began to feel the results. She was quite listless for two days. That has improved, but she is still very low on energy and is sleeping quite a bit. Remarkably, she now has no pain. She is taking no pain medication at all! This is within a week of her asking for more pain medication within two hours of having taken a 4-hour dose. I'm not sure what to think of this development, but am very grateful for it. Her low energy level bothers her because there are things she would like to do but just does not feel like it. Today, I suggested that she call someone on the phone just for a short conversation, but she rejected that idea. She says "I just don't feel up to it."

This week will be busy. Sheila has an appointment to see her surgeon on Monday and is having her children come to the house on Friday evening for a small birthday gathering for Allan and Connie, whose birthdays are just weeks apart in late April, early May. I'm leaving for a visit with my family in Pennsylvania on Thursday and will be gone until Sunday.

The mail continues to be a highlight of each day. Your faithfulness in this regard is so much appreciated and means so much to Sheila. And it is very encouraging for me to observe. Thank you very much.

Until next time!

Again, we were making arrangements for coverage while I went away for a visit to family, partly for a break and partly for a late celebration of my mother's birthday. We had to arrange for the nurses to come in to do the hook-ups since Connie and Mark were not available to handle those duties. Mark came and slept at the house at night so Sheila wouldn't be alone, so that was helpful.

I was pleasantly surprised by her announcement that she wanted to go to church with me. I had been going every week since this all began. It provided an opportunity to update people on how things were going during conversation before and after church. I drew a crowd. So many people loved and missed Sheila there. My church attendance was also necessary for my personal strength. I cannot articulate anything specific that sustained me. I just needed to be in that community surrounded by the people who I knew would help us in an instant if we needed it. Such is the reality of the presence of God for me.

Sheila told me that she didn't think she had the stamina to endure a lot of greetings and questions about her well-being, but that she really wanted to go to church. So we devised a strategy to go late and leave early.

As we walked up the ramp toward the church door, Sheila was to my right. We were walking along slowly, talking about nothing much, when I felt her hand reach for mine. Her grip was strong and she was not unsteady on her feet at all. I think she just wanted me to stay close. We walked hand in hand into the church narthex and there was the choir all lined up ready to process into the sanctuary.

Someone spotted her and said, "Sheila's here!" There was a momentary pause before the entire group of about twenty people broke into applause.

I'm sure the people in the sanctuary had to wonder about the commotion behind them. Sheila walked toward the front of the lined-up choir members and she was immediately engulfed in hugs and expressions of joy at her appearance. It was very heart-warming to see their sincere delight at her presence.

Never before and never since have I received an ovation for going to church.

5-11-08

Sheila had a pretty good week since I last wrote. She went to church, went to the doctor, had a small birthday party for two of her children, and had a good time while I was away visiting my family in Pennsylvania.

Last Sunday morning, Sheila woke up feeling pretty good and decided to go to church. She had been uncomfortable sitting on the hard pew when she attended before, so I went prepared this time with a cushion that I knew was comfortable for her. But toward the end of the service, she motioned to me that she wanted to leave. When we got outside, she explained that her back was bothering her as she sat there. So, if she feels up to attending again, we will make provision for a more comfortable seating arrangement for her. But we had a nice little outing anyway, stopping for coffee at McDonald's after we left church and it felt good.

On Monday, Sheila had an appointment with her surgeon, Dr. Chambers. It was a routine follow-up as far as Sheila and the doctor were concerned, but I had an agenda. I wanted to talk to him about the ordeal of the ER to see if there is some way to avoid that in the future, should the G-Tube need attention again. He's very attentive to Sheila and was extremely positive about her condition, telling her she looked really good, that he thought her abdomen felt good, that our care of the G-tube skin area was "excellent" (I was proud).

When the two of them had finished with their interaction, I asked him if we had done anything that would have contributed to the failure of the G-tube which resulted in the prolonged ER visit. No, lots of things can cause such failures, but if we have problems again, he had two suggestions. One is that we should always try to keep the tube in. If it comes out, we need to stick it back in, because, if the passageway closes up, it would require "a procedure" to reestablish it. OK, I was reassured that nothing about my care of the tube had contributed to the failure and I thought that we should be able to keep the thing in there.

I must say that I began to get a bit nervous when he seemed to talk himself into the idea that we should have a spare "Foley Kit" just in case the current tube comes out. He began to explain how to insert the new tube, push slightly (but not too much), inflate the "balloon" with saline (but not too much), and pull until there was resistance (you guessed it—not too much)—all this so the passageway can be maintained because it can close in several hours. His second suggestion was that we should call him if we have problems in the future and he can maybe expedite things in the ER a bit. I like that second option the best! But he insisted on running over to the ER on our way out to secure his trusty "Foley Kit" for us to bring home.

Dr. Chambers was also interested in whether Sheila is drinking anything. He seemed pleased that she is enjoying fruit juices occasionally. Then he said, "I think you could also try ice cream or milk shakes. No food, but you could try dairy products. Go to Dairy Queen two or three times a week." YESS!! Sheila would have to have company, of course. We can't have her drinking alone. So I keep telling her that the doctor has ordered us to Dairy Queen. She, unfortunately, doesn't like ice cream very much (I think someone dropped her on her head when she was little and damaged the ice cream-loving area of her brain), so we haven't really done it. But I keep lobbying.

The remainder of the week was fairly routine in terms of Sheila's condition. She continues to experience some nausea and we keep the pink tubs handy. It's hard to know what triggers that and I feel very frustrated by it because I want to give her something to relieve it. We're properly using all of the medication that the oncologist has prescribed, but I think some adjustment may be needed. She's already sick enough without that uncomfortable experience every two or three days.

I guess the birthday party was a great success. I missed it because I was in Pennsylvania, but reviews from the attendees I've talked with are very positive. I really appreciate that Sheila's children provided coverage here while I was away. It's obvious that they took very good care of her and I enjoyed my stay in Pennsylvania.

The second chemo treatment is scheduled for this week, on Wednesday. Sheila has already had one set of follow-up blood tests and will have two more this week prior to the treatment. So if all looks good, they will proceed, as far as we know. The good news is that she's tolerated the first one well enough to be ready for the second, at least from an energy level standpoint. She continues to tire easily and battles the nausea, but otherwise has had few adverse side effects, so that is relatively positive. And, to my eternal amazement, she is still taking no pain medication at all. I'm eager to see what Dr. Cohn, the gynecological oncologist, thinks when he sees her after the chemo treatment.

The treatment itself is administered through the same PICC line in her arm that I use for her feeding. It takes about an hour and she will see Dr. Cohn after the treatment is over. So she will spend a good part of Wednesday getting ready to go, traveling to the office, receiving the treatment, seeing the doctor, and getting home. I'll have one tired patient at the end of that day! But Sheila never complains and has a very cooperative attitude about all of this. Very impressive.

The animals and I are glad to report no incidents of any note this past week. Sometimes a typical routine is a great blessing, it seems to me. So we're grateful for that and many other things, including the dedicated and compassionate care of the various medical professionals who are tending to Sheila. And we're humbled that so many of you express a desire to "do something" for us. Your cards and prayers are exactly what we need and your faithful attention in that way has been most sustaining. If you can, we would ask that you continue to support us in this way. And thank you for all that you have already done.

I was so impressed by Dr. Chambers. He seemed to genuinely care about Sheila's recovery. He listened to her and to me, said encouraging things to her, complimented her on how well she was doing, and encouraged her visits with Dr. Cohn. I appreciated his attention to my concerns about managing the tube. I have never known a doctor to interrupt his day to walk with us to the exit of his office building, literally run across the parking lot, and run back toward where we were waiting, happily waiving a pack of medical supplies he had instantly procured from the adjacent ER facility. He handed them over to me with great satisfaction and sincerely wished Sheila well until he'd see her again.

Privately I wanted to get Sheila home because I knew that the effort to make the trip and interact with him was tiring her. And I was doubting that his efforts would be helpful because I would be unlikely to properly use the materials anyway. His confidence was misplaced, I was pretty sure.

5-18-08

This week Sheila experienced the failure of her PICC line, a chemo treatment, an aborted blood transfusion, a successful blood transfusion, and "occupational therapy" as designed by Nurse Ratchet.

Things started off pretty well, as I remember. The week became interesting at 5:30 a.m. on Wednesday, the day of the scheduled chemo treatment. Sheila called me (unusual these days, so I knew something was up) and when I arrived at her bedside, she advised that her PICC line was leaking. Once before we had experienced a leak because I had improperly attached it, but that seemed to be an unlikely cause this time because it had been running for 13 hours by the time this complication was discovered.

Upon inspection, I could see that the connection was not the problem. Something appeared to be wrong within the line mechanism itself. Plan A was to call the nurse on call. They are very prompt with their return calls, so we did not wait long. As this was unfolding, I was already formulating my "resistance speech" if any trip to the ER was suggested. I was not at all inclined to take Sheila to the ER for an interminable wait for the PICC line specialist, who once had to come from West Virginia (when Sheila was in the hospital). And she would miss the chemo treatment while sitting in the ER.

The nurse listened to my description of the problem and said, "That's not something we can come out and fix. You need the PICC line specialist. I suggest you take her to the ER." I resisted the urge to say something unkind. After all, this woman was no doubt awakened from her sleep and did not need to listen to me being snide. We needed plan B. The nurse had no other suggestions, understandably, and I politely (from my perspective, anyway) ended that conversation.

Sheila, by this time, was beginning to plan her wardrobe for the day and was giving some thought to how she was going to get her hair to look good for whatever the day's events would turn out to be. I interrupted her planning to suggest that we call Dr. Chambers despite the fact that this problem was not a G-tube problem. Since he had just offered to help by-pass the ER in case the tube was a problem, I thought he might be willing to assist with this situation. So Sheila called his pager. Sure enough, he called back very shortly thereafter, listened to the issue, and told her he'd see if he could confirm the presence of a PICC line specialist in the hospital. He told her it would be 30 minutes or so before she'd hear anything. Plan B was unfolding relatively well, I thought.

Then, Sheila announced that Dr. Chambers, who's affiliated with Mt. Carmel Hospitals, also suggested the possibility of someone at OSU replacing the line. Oh, my; we now had a Plan C. We talked about calling Dr. Cohn's office staff to discuss options there. About this time, Dr. Chambers called back to tell Sheila that he did not locate the PICC line specialist, but wanted her to know that he had not forgotten about her. I tell you, even though the medical care system is profoundly frustrating, the people who work in it are outstanding, if our experience is any indication. Anyway, it was too early to call Dr. Cohn's office. At this point, I took a shower, Sheila went back to planning her grooming activities for the day, and Sheila's son Mark came through the door because he was on duty for the day.

As it turned out, it was all better than it might have been. Through Dr. Chambers, arrangements were made for Sheila to see the PICC line specialist at Mt. Carmel after her chemo treatment. So they went to the treatment at Dr. Cohn's office and then to an outpatient facility at Mt. Carmel where the PICC line malfunction was confirmed and a new one inserted. So the patient was about done in when they finally got home. But her hair looked great.

Sheila reported that Dr. Cohn was pleased with her condition other than her red blood cell count. It was almost so low as to prevent the chemo treatment, but he decided to go ahead anyway. He ordered two pints of blood, to be infused at the ICC facility at OSU on Thursday. All was well on Wednesday evening after the chemo treatment until Ernie the cat ventured into territory where he doesn't belong and knocked over Sheila's pill container that we had just filled with her post-chemo medications. At that moment, I almost became a dog person.

Mark was on call again on Thursday, so he took Sheila to OSU for her scheduled appointment at noon for the blood transfusion. But, after they arrived, they were told that Sheila's blood was not easy to match and they might not have it until 4:00 p.m. and then it would take four hours to infuse. Why nobody knew this in time to save the trip in there is beyond me. So that mission was aborted and rescheduled for Friday.

Connie was here Friday and took Sheila to OSU, where the transfusion went as expected. I picked her up on my way home from Cleveland where I had been on business and we stopped at Dairy Queen, just as the doctor ordered. It was great. Sheila has been feeling good these past few days. We needed the pink tub one time, but the Dairy Queen treat was long gone by then, thank goodness. I'm angling for a return trip tomorrow, so want to avoid any suggestion that the Dairy Queen trips contribute to nausea.

Today was an especially good day. Sheila felt able to do several household tasks, and when I suggested that she empty the dishwasher, she informed me that she did not want too much of "Nurse Ratchet's occupational therapy." I promptly reminded her that she's totally dependent on "Nurse Ratchet" for her daily feeding, so too much antagonism would not be in her best interest.

If this post-chemo process resembles the last one, Sheila's still in for a day or two of feeling listless. The last time it was days six and seven, which would be Tuesday and Wednesday of this week. It may be that the transfusion will mute that reaction, so we can hope for that. Dr. Cohn has encouraged Sheila to eat pudding and broth or something else that's soft. So she's trying that very carefully at this point. I would be absolutely thrilled to relinquish my "hooker" job because her digestive system begins to respond well to food.

I continue to be so thankful that Sheila receives mail from well-wishers every day. It really means a lot. Your prayer support is evident to us as we see reasons to be thankful and feel the strength of God's presence with us in this. Thank you for everything you are doing to help us.

Until next time.

I was feeling like we were making some progress. Sheila was tolerating the treatments as well as might be expected and Dr. Cohn inspired so much confidence. The daily medical routines were our new way of life. I was beginning to think about a day when we might restore the rest of our former routines.

I was especially pleased when Sheila stopped her dishwasher duties one day and looked out the kitchen window for quite a while. I wondered what she was thinking, but didn't interrupt her thoughts. I just watched her. When she turned around she said, "I just love to watch those finches." I loved to see her enjoying them and was glad that I had kept the feeder full. Just a few short weeks prior, she didn't have the energy to stand there, not to mention the energy to watch birds for a while.

5-25-08

Sheila had a pretty good week this past week and the animals and I caused no trouble at all, I'm happy to report. In fact, things were nearly routine around here for a change.

As predicted, Sheila did feel listless and ill for several days mid-week. I think it was the post-chemo impact hitting her. The good thing is, she bounces back and keeps going and even though she felt like it, she did not have to use the pink tub.

Sheila went to church last week and is planning to go this morning. Yesterday we made a visit to the graves of her parents, Allan, and sister-in-law Barbara. We had a very pleasant drive out there, placed flowers on the graves, and then stopped at Wendy's so Sheila could try the new strawberry frosty milk shake. Strawberry is her favorite flavor and she's rather expert at assessing strawberry flavored things, having taste tested most anything she can get her hands on. She pronounced the Wendy's effort to be "a bit too artificial. They tried too hard." I stuck with the good old chocolate frosty. I thought mine was fine.

Sheila also had a visit from a former neighbor who was in town. He's 92 years old and had not been by his former home since he sold it to move in with his children in Cleveland several years ago. She was glad to see him but was very tired afterward, even though he was here for only about an hour. So she is still limiting visitors until she regains more strength. It's hard to know when that might happen with the ongoing chemo creating a constant drain.

You may recall that one of the doctor's orders was for her to try to eat puddings and ice cream. She's been working on that and enjoys the puddings. She's also drinking fruit juices, hot tea, and her daily Starbucks Frappuccino, a concoction newly introduced to her by daughter Connie. It is now a regular entry on the store list each week. I'm very glad that Sheila is enjoying the intake of these things, but I believe the truth is that her digestive system is not working any better than it has since the first of the year. Most all of what she takes in just flows right back out through the G-tube. However, if she enjoys consuming, I'll provide whatever she wants. This makes her feel less like a sick person, I think. And, who knows, maybe one day her digestion processes will resume.

I think that's all the news from our corner of the world. Sheila commented to me again this week about how much she appreciates the cards and prayers of her friends and relatives. Her contact with people has to be so limited right now that the mail becomes a highlight of each day. Thank you so much for your continued attention to her in this way. It's helping her! And we appreciate it very much.

Ever since I had lived with her, I observed Sheila's dedication to visiting the cemetery just before Memorial Day. She took flowers to Allan's grave and those of her parents and sister-in-law. So I was not surprised when she mentioned a cemetery visit. I offered to buy the flowers and go to the cemetery for her, but she said she felt well enough to go along, so we got in the car for a little venture. I had taken the day off so we could spend some time together. It was a great day weather-wise and Sheila was pleased to feel up to the trip.

We stopped first to buy flowers. I received very specific instructions on the size of the flowers, color, and variety. One presentation had to be a small bouquet to attach to Barbara's crypt, another, a potted plant. She inspected my purchases carefully when I returned to the car and I was pleased to receive her approval. I was also trying to keep things moving along because I wasn't sure how much stamina she would have, despite her ambitious intentions.

As we drove out to the cemetery, we talked mostly about her parents, and about how nice it was to be out together for a while. We seemed like normal people, not people who lived with nightly IV hook-ups and baby monitors and chemo treatments. At the cemetery, we drove first to Allan's grave, quite near where Sheila's parents are buried. She wanted to get out of the car and walk to the graves, a short distance. She supervised my placement of the flowers, talked about how visiting the cemetery was an obligation and not a place of emotional connection for her, and we got back into the car

Our final stop was near Barbara's crypt, with Sheila explaining that since Steve was so far away, she felt that she should take time to remember Barbara for him on Memorial Day. She got out of the car again and made her way to the crypt. She was making me a bit nervous because I was so concerned for her ability to do this. But she plowed on and seemed pleased by what had been accomplished. I didn't relate well to the cemetery decorating commitment, but wanted to support whatever she felt like doing.

As we left, I reminded her that the intake of dairy products had been ordered by the doctor, so perhaps we should fill a prescription, so to speak. There had been no tears or moments of lament or sadness at the cemetery, but I thought we could use an upbeat tone as we made our way home. There was a Wendy's in a perfect location. The biggest pleasure for me was that Sheila enjoyed it.

5-31-08

Sheila's had a good week. She still tires easily and has little stamina, but is working to expand her activities around the house to spaces beyond her chair in the family room and her bed in the dining room. She goes upstairs each day for her shower, occasionally makes a greeting card on the computer, and usually assists with the laundry.

Her eating situation is unchanged. She enjoys the intake of various juices, teas, coffees, puddings, and ice cream. But she doesn't really digest much of it from what we can tell. It mostly comes back out her G-tube. One day this week, she wanted to try drinking and eating pudding while the tube was clamped off. She was able to tolerate that for several hours, but then needed relief. And it was obvious from the activity in the tube when we reconnected it that she had not digested much. So we are hopeful that upcoming treatments will result in more progress with this situation.

Sheila is able to attend church and has received a few extended family visitors, but still gets very tired after those events. It's hard to make progress when she has a chemo treatment every three weeks that slows her down. She just gets to feeling stronger when it's time for another treatment.

Speaking of treatments, she is scheduled for her next one on Thursday June 5. She will receive the chemotherapy via her IV and then see the doctor. I know she is interested to learn the results of her blood tests and to talk with him in general about her condition. He is very committed to doing everything possible to improve her quality of life. He is encouraging her to try to eat puddings and ice creams with the G-tube clamped off. It will be interesting to see what he thinks of the fact that she's trying, but her digestive system does not seem to be responding yet.

The animals and I have done well this week, too. Ernie the cat has really become Sheila's buddy. He sits on her lap each day now and she likes his company. Unfortunately, he has also become fascinated by the IV lines, which have, from a cat's perspective, wonderful little things dangling from them. He sneaks up to her chair when nobody is paying attention and whacks at those things, startling Sheila into a yelp, prompting the dog to want to either rescue someone or engage in the fun, and inspiring me to make a fool of myself trying to whack Ernie. If anyone was watching us at those moments, they would call the social services and animal control people to rescue all of us.

When I asked Sheila what I should say in this note, she said "Tell them I have a treatment this week, I'm working on getting better, and I feel their prayers."

There you have it!

6-7-08

Sheila had an up and down week, the animals and I are fine, and there is encouraging news from the oncologist this week.

The home health care nurses continue to reinforce the doctors' instructions for Sheila to try to eat things that are easy to digest. They remind her that her digestive system has not been doing anything for six months, so it needs to be "retrained" by introducing food gradually. And if the system resists, she's supposed to keep trying. Easy for them to say.

So this week, Sheila ate applesauce and visited the pink tub several hours later. The next day she had a strawberry sundae. Pink tub several hours later. The day after that, she had soup. Pink tub several hours later. I'm amazed at her ability to keep trying. She has enormous mental strength through all of this, from my perspective, and her persistence with this eating process is prime evidence.

Fortunately, we have developed a highly choreographed routine around the pink tub visits. After Sheila announces the need to use it, she grabs the tub (we always have one close at hand), I head for the bathroom to get a cool washcloth for the back of her neck (a technique picked up from the nurses in the hospital that makes her feel much better), make sure she has Kleenex at hand, and get the spare tub so we can swap at the appropriate time. One day, the poor dog happened to be in the room and she was most interested in the unfolding events and accompanying activities, took two steps toward Sheila and decided that was far enough, and quickly retreated to a spot on the hearth out of the way. Sheila laughed and noted, "Hildey doesn't want any part of this!"

After three days of that, it was time for the doctor visit. I had taken the day off, so we planned a leisurely start to the day because the appointment was not until 12:30. But Sheila had a very rough night.

Her pain returned and she was very uncomfortable for most of the night. I was administering pain medication and praying for relief and she finally fell asleep for a while; however, she did not feel well all morning. When we got to the parking lot of the doctor's office, she said, "I'm going to throw up" and reached for the ever-present pink tub. Sure enough, she did. And the highly choreographed routine was out the window. I'm sitting there thinking, "What am I going to do with the pink tub contents?" while Sheila was apologizing for throwing up and expressing concern about being late for her appointment. Ever practical, I said "Don't worry; they won't start your chemo treatment without you."

Needless to say, we improvised the pink tub routine (I made mental notes of new supplies that must be added to our stash of stuff in the car in case of a repeat performance) and got Sheila into the doctor's office. This is where things started looking up.

The doctor has been tracking a blood factor that suggests the presence of cancer. "Normal" readings are 10-12. Sheila's was 432 before her first chemo treatment. On Thursday, he told her it had been over 700 in the weeks since, but in the latest test, it was 40. This is extremely positive news, very pleasing for the doctor to tell her, and most encouraging for Sheila to hear. Apparently his attitude about her situation is very positive. She said to me, "I think he thinks he can make me better."

When she told him about the pain and nausea in the days immediately preceding her visit, he told her that such occurrences are not uncommon in his patients. He called it "anticipatory anxiety-induced pain and nausea" and told her it's not at all uncommon for people to throw up in the parking lot of the office. He added, "I'm very careful about where I walk out there." That really made her laugh when she re-told that to me.

He is also encouraging her to resume as many of her regular activities as possible. He wants her to walk, do small things around the house, and even take a short trip this summer. When I heard that, I told her I'd take her anywhere she wants to go, make a list of household chores for her to do, and walk with her whenever she felt like going. And I know that her other "attendants" who are here during the day are doing the same thing.

So we are very thankful for the apparent progress against the cancer and hopeful that the digestive system will begin to respond. Progress with eating is the biggest thing. The daily need for 16 hours of IV feeding and the constant presence of the G-tube are compromising Sheila's quality of life right now. She has spent some time in the kitchen this week doing small things despite feeling pretty "weak and wrung out" in the two days since the treatment. That usually continues for about a week, so she will be somewhat under the weather for most of the coming week.

She continues to find joy and encouragement in your cards and notes that arrive each day. Walking to the mailbox is a highlight of each day. Sheila is also quite sure that your faithful prayers are very much contributing to her positive progress. Thank you and thank God.

When I got home from the office on Thursday, I knew it had not been a good day. Mark was with his mother and Sheila was sitting in her chair, wearing the same clothes she had been wearing in the morning.

"How was your day?" I asked as I studied her while trying to look like I wasn't.

"I didn't feel very well today. I didn't even go upstairs for my shower."

Mark confirmed that she had been a bit tired. And shortly thereafter, he left and I began preparations to connect the IV. We tried to get that done as soon as I got home because such timing allowed for earlier unhooking the next morning.

I got the IV connected, went upstairs to change clothes, and found Sheila looking very bad when I got back down the steps. She began to shiver and I was now on full alert. I wrapped her up in a blanket and she said something nonsensical to me. I never heard something like that from a person before. She looked at me and knew she hadn't made sense, but couldn't speak much at all.

OK, we're not messing with this. I called the telephone number provided by Dr. Cohn's office and asked for the resident on call, as instructed. When I talked to the resident and described the situation, her reaction was immediate. She really got my attention when she said, "Sepsis is very serious. Tell her she could die if we don't treat her in time."

There was no way I was telling Sheila she might die, but there was also no way she was going to persuade me to take her to the ER in a car. She needed the pros this time.

On the way to the hospital in a major thunderstorm, I called Connie, updated her, and asked her to call her brothers. I went racing into that ER, trying to control my emotions and feeling amazed at how quickly things had gone bad.

6-13-08

We have breaking news and it's not good. Sheila was hospitalized this evening after a very hard day of feeling ill and visiting with the pink tub multiple times. That would have been manageable but things changed early in the evening when she experienced a sudden onset of severe chills. I could tell that her condition was more than I could manage, so I persuaded her that we needed to contact the oncology resident on call for guidance.

Those folks do respond to calls very quickly, and I said only, "She's having chills that came on all of a sudden" and the doctor said "We need to see her" before I could explain anything else. I knew Sheila would resist going to the hospital and that she would resist going in the emergency vehicle. I asked the doctor to tell me what she was worried about and whether it would expedite things if Sheila went to the hospital via a car or the squad. The doctor said " Tell her I'm worried about sepsis (and something else unpronounceable that I forget) and tell her that you should not be driving her around when it's shortly after rush hour and it's raining so hard up here I can hardly hear you when you talk. Please call me back after you decide what you're doing." Good plan.

As predicted, Sheila resisted and I made my pitch. I became increasingly insistent during this brief debate because the more I observed her, the more sure I was that we needed help and that I should hand her off to professional people who could tend to her properly. I called 911 and began to do the things they prompt you to do even before they reviewed the list with me (unlock the door, put animals away, get a list of medications ready, call us back if she stops breathing).

As the EMTs began their interview and examination of Sheila, she provided some strange answers to their questions, which was a continuation of her speech patterns when she and I were talking while waiting for them to arrive. So on top of the chills, we now had Sheila experiencing difficulty expressing herself properly, speaking nonsense words or saying things that were out of context. My anxiety level doubled. And we were soon off to the races.

No need for long stories about the typical ordeal of an ER visit. They did usher her into a private room with a door that closed and she received relatively prompt attention. Sheila's temperature is only slightly elevated, her white blood cell count is "pretty good," and she showed signs of dehydration. So they administered antibiotics, anti-nausea medications, and additional fluids right away and told us that she would be in the hospital for several days. When I asked how worried we should be, several doctors and nurses said, "We are always very concerned when a chemo patient has a fever that might suggest an infection. We will know more in a few days as we watch how she responds to treatment and after more testing to confirm what we're dealing with."

They finally gave Sheila enough medication that she was completely sacked out when I left, to the point where she could not wake up to answer the doctor's questions when she came back in several times later in the evening. They were moving Sheila to a "step down" unit after ruling out the need for ICU. They definitely don't want her on a regular floor because of the concern about exposure to infection. So visitations will be limited to her children and she should not receive flowers or gifts of any kind.

This is a disappointing setback and a potentially serious situation, as I understand things. It all depends how Sheila responds to the treatment provided during the next few days. I will do my best to provide updates as things unfold. Your continued prayers for us are very much needed at this time.

I sat in that freezing cold ER room and watched the doctors tend to my very sick friend. They quickly administered some drugs and took blood. Whatever they did knocked her out. The resident wanted a medical history and Sheila couldn't provide it. Fortunately, I was able to do it easily, having lived through it with her for the past twelve years. Again, I wondered what happened for people who had nobody with them at the hospital.

I just sat there. I couldn't leave her. I wanted more information about a plan for further treatment and the nurses kept telling me that the oncology resident from Dr. Cohn's service was coming. I wasn't leaving until I spoke to that person.

Minutes turned into hours. I had taken to pacing the halls, both to try to calm myself and to stay warm. The resident finally arrived around midnight, noted that I was medical POA, reviewed Sheila's chart, and explained the plan assuming an infection, but further tests would be needed to be certain. She was hopeful for a positive response. Then she asked a question that I had not been asked before and that nearly broke me, "If she does not respond and her condition worsens, what are her wishes? What do you want us to do?"

I stared at her. My eyes started filling with tears. I was dead tired, discouraged, cold, and weak. I knew the answer, but could not speak for a moment. The resident stopped writing on the chart and looked at me kindly. "I know it's hard. We are hopeful that she will respond. But I have to ask, so we are clear about what to do in case something goes bad here overnight."

The best I could do was nod to her that I understood the reason for the question. She waited patiently for my response. I finally choked out the words I knew I had to say, but that I could hardly face at that moment, "Let her go."

She made a note in the chart, thanked me, and excused herself with assurance to me that they would take good care of Sheila.

I just sat there. This was the first time I had to confront the reality of Sheila's death as an imminent possibility, not a distant maybe. I looked at her on that ER gurney, zonked out, full of drugs, tube connecting her to her nutrition and tube discharging excess fluids, and I felt sad and tired. And I wanted her to rally and get better more than I ever wanted anything ever. But there was nothing I could do to make it happen.

I finally left and made my way to the parking garage where I had left my car. It was too late for any attendants to be in the booth, so I drove up to the lowered gate and read the instructions wearily. "Between midnight and 6:00 a.m. please insert credit card to pay and release the gate." Right. I didn't care how much they would charge; I just wanted to get out of there. I followed the instructions and nothing happened. I re-read the instructions and followed the process again. Nothing happened. I was locked in the parking garage at OSU hospital at 1:00 a.m. and I was in no mood to be tolerant. I noticed a button to summon security. I pushed it. A man's voice answered and asked me what I needed.

I explained my predicament as patiently as I could.

"Which garage are you in?"

"I have no idea. It's the one across from the hospital."

"Tenth Avenue, Canon Drive, or the Main Garage?"

Seriously? I was exceedingly close to ending this conversation, backing my car up, and driving right through that little gate and racing home. I didn't care about damage to my car or the consequences of my actions or anything else. I was just completely done.

"I think it's Canon Drive, but I'm not sure." I said, having located a reserve of strength from an unknown place so I could stay engaged with this fellow who really was trying to help me.

"Is there a green sign on the building across from you?"

"Yes"

"I'll get there as soon as I can, ma'am."

I knew that whenever he got there would not be soon enough. I tried to settle myself. I tried to think of something other than Sheila lying in the ER room all alone in serious condition. I tried not to feel guilty about leaving her. I tried to tell myself that if she recovered, she would need me and I had to rest. I tried to remind myself that if I had stayed, she wouldn't even know I was there. I tried not to scream or cry. I really wanted to plow through that gate.

The security guy arrived and apologized for the "trouble," explaining that there were recent problems with the gating system in the parking garages after hours.

"So why not just put the gates up and allow everyone to leave?" I wondered, but didn't care enough to ask.

I drove home feeling empty and alone. I got home at around 1:30, knowing I had to make an appearance at the office the next day. A special event was going on and my absence would be noticeable. I owed it to my group to get there. I didn't sleep much that night.

6-15-08

The past 48 hours have been quite eventful, but the good news is that Sheila has improved. It turns out that her condition was life-threatening, she spent the night in the ER on Thursday and doesn't remember it (thank goodness!), and I was admonished by a four-year-old on my dog obedience techniques. Once again, we'll go in order.

When I left the ER on Thursday night, the plan was for Sheila's abdomen to be scanned (without use of the troublesome stuff they usually try to make her drink that she resists and then "gives back") and for her to be admitted to a room where she could be watched carefully.

At 7:00 a.m. Friday, I called the hospital to check on her condition and her location. I was surprised when I was told that "She's still in the ER." I said that couldn't be, but after multiple calls and transfers to various departments within the hospital, I finally reached a helpful nurse in the ER who even put Sheila on the phone. So I had to believe she was still in the ER. But she didn't sound good and the nurse said they had not moved her because there were no beds available. We needed a plan.

Enter Annabelle, the nurse affiliated with Dr. Cohn's office who had saved the day at least once previously. I called her office even though it was before hours, and left a message indicating my concern about Sheila being in the ER all night, including a suggestion that it might be appropriate to move her to Mt. Carmel. Sure enough, Annabelle checked into everything and called me back to say that the hospital was on a "level 2 staffing alert, and Mt. Carmel's on a level 3." Translation: There were no beds in the hospitals and Mt. Carmel's situation was worse than OSU's. I knew that Sheila really wanted to be at OSU, so my threat was an empty one, but it made me feel like I was at least letting these folks know that someone was looking out for her well-being.

Annabelle assured me that they thought a bed would open up later in the day, the ER nurses were top notch and would provide very attentive care, and things would work out. But I had little information on Sheila's condition at that point and I didn't like that. Annabelle emphatically suggested that I wait until the afternoon to come to the hospital (she probably envisioned a wild woman charging in there causing **nothing** constructive to occur), so I reluctantly planned accordingly and updated Sheila's children.

When I found Sheila on Friday afternoon, she was settled into her room, was receiving massive doses of medications, and was finally resting comfortably, from what I could tell. Her nurse explained that they were treating her for infection, her temperature was over 102, the nausea was subsiding, her vital signs were stable but not quite what they wanted them to be, and she needed rest. I could tell by looking at her that she was very ill. I asked the nurse how we could get information directly from the doctors and learned that we should be at the hospital on Saturday morning between 8:00 and 10:00 a.m. when they would be making rounds. So I sat and watched the monitors for a few hours, updated the kids again, and came home.

This morning when I arrived, I could tell immediately that Sheila was better. She looked better, was talkative, and was interested in the headlines in the morning paper. Dr. Cohn himself and a small entourage arrived as planned around 9:30 and he said; "Sheila, how nice of you to come to the hospital to see me. This way, I don't have to put on a tie and my office attire to see you!" After a good laugh with everyone (Sheila's daughter and son-in law were there, too), he said, "We're treating you for sepsis. This condition causes your heart rate to go up, your blood pressure to go down, and can kill you. But we think we have it under control now." That got everyone's attention.

Later, Sheila said, "That's what got the puppet guy." It didn't take us too long to translate her comment as meaning what caused the death of Puppeteer Jim Hensen, creator of the Muppets. Sobering thought.

Dr. Cohn went on to explain that this condition is a bacterial infection in the blood, the cause of which is uncertain. With as many devices as Sheila has needed to use, there are multiple possibilities. One prime likelihood is the PICC line we use to feed her. He said they were going to take it out, but that her nutrition would be OK for a few weeks. They are also treating her for a bladder infection, so she is receiving large amounts of antibiotics right now. Her temperature and vital signs are back to normal.

The doctor also reported that the scan of Sheila's belly showed "no change." Thus, it seems that, despite the encouraging blood test results recently, the cancer remains a concern and there is no evidence of a return to normal functioning in her digestive system. He indicated that they would continue to treat Sheila and strive to improve her quality of life.

I spoke with Sheila on the phone this evening and she's sounding pretty good. She did not have to experience "tray envy" when everyone else received something at meal time because they brought her what she asked for, potato soup and yogurt. She said she ate a little bit of it. It's probably going right out the G-tube, but she enjoys it on the way down, so that's the important thing right now from my perspective.

This afternoon, Hildey and I went for a walk in the park. As we were passing by the lake, a little girl whose family was fishing from the dock spotted us coming and immediately ran to greet Hildey. (The dog is the attraction in the park, Sheila is the attraction in church. I'm mostly invisible when I'm with either of them.) As the child approached, I encouraged Hildey to stop, and the little girl, who obviously has spent time around dogs, asked if the dog was a boy or a girl and if she could pet her. When I said yes, I, in my most commanding dog-instruction voice said, "Hildey, sit." As the dog continued to prance around with excitement at the meeting of a new friend, the child said, "No, you have to give her a treat to make her sit down. Don't you have a treat?" Humbled, I said "No" and wanted to add, "I'm a cat person and no self-respecting cat would be glad to greet a totally strange child, not to mention respond positively to a command, treat or not." But I didn't. I "made nice" with the little girl and soon prompted Hildey to move along.

Back to Sheila. Next steps are uncertain at this point. I believe she will remain in the hospital under careful watch until they are completely sure that the crisis has passed. Your continued cards, thoughts, and prayers will be most helpful as we navigate through the next steps on this journey. Thank you very much for your faithful attention to us. It's difficult to express how much it means.

That early morning phone call was discouraging, except that at least Sheila had survived the night. I made one call to Connie to update the family. I had to go to the office for a while, so got myself together in the morning and went, trying to hide my physical and emotional exhaustion. Fortunately, the special event was casual, I made proper appearances, acted like I was enjoying my team's company, and then took one of my managers aside and explained that I was leaving to go to the hospital. I also said something to my boss on the way out so she knew why I was leaving early.

When I got to OSU that afternoon, I was tired and annoyed that Sheila had spent the night in the ER. I knew this was not a good attitude to have when intending to be a source of positive energy for a loved one but I couldn't stay away. If Sheila was awake, I wanted her to know that someone was there with her. I nominated myself, despite not being at my best. She was still so sick. I could see that. I walked into her room as the staff was transferring her to a regular bed. She had obviously just arrived from the ER.

I was incensed when I saw the daughter of a friend of Sheila's, a technician who worked in another area of the hospital, standing there in the room. She had no reason to be present, regardless of her intentions and it was inappropriate for her to have inserted herself into this situation. Sheila had repeatedly expressed a desire for privacy as she worked to recover and even her children at this moment had not yet received updated information on their mother's condition. Seeing this person, who did not belong in Sheila's room under any circumstance, inflamed my every protective and assertive instinct on behalf of my helpless friend.

A nurse who had introduced himself as Sheila's primary nurse was standing watching as others, including the intruder, tended to Sheila. I tapped him on the shoulder, motioned for him to follow me, and walked back out of the room. "I am Sheila's housemate and medical power of attorney. I am asking you as nicely as I can manage right now to assure me that Marilyn will be asked to leave that room immediately. She thinks she is a close friend. She is not. Sheila has been private about her illness in terms of visitors. Most certainly this technician should not be privy to the condition of this patient. She is not welcome now and she will not be welcome in the future. I will not speak to her nicely if I try to deliver that message right now. I am asking you to take care of it for us." I looked at him with a face that quite clearly told him I was not kidding.

I always tried to control my facial expressions in Sheila's presence so I exuded calm and control. At this moment, however, there was no question that I was angry and highly motivated to change the reality of what was going on in that room. To his credit, the nurse listened to me closely, studied my face for just a moment, and said, "I understand. I will take care of this for you." He then went back into Sheila's room.

I walked away. The staff was getting her settled and I needed to collect myself. I was exhausted and alone and scared. I found a seat in a little waiting area near the nurse's station, sat down, and allowed myself a few trickles of tears. I just sat there with my head down, trying to find a way to collect myself enough to get back to the mission at hand: finding out what Sheila's condition was and what the treatment plan was.

Just a few moments later, Marilyn sat down beside me, put her arm around me, and began a series of utterances that she thought were comforting. I am not proud to say that I barely acknowledged her presence, kept my head down, nodded occasionally, and desperately wanted her to leave me alone. I never even looked at her as she got up to leave, but fortunately for her I didn't say what I was thinking. I was finished with being angry before she even sat down. I just wanted to find the energy to go tend to Sheila.

Again, Sheila was mostly uncommunicative. She acknowledged my presence initially when I got into her room, and then quickly settled into a deep sleep. My information came from the nurse, who was wonderful and assured me that Sheila would be monitored closely and that I would be contacted if her condition changed. He urged me to go home and get some rest. The poor guy probably recognized a woman who was working on her last nerve. But I had to be there for a while, so I just sat again and thought how glad I was that Sheila had survived the night. I also began to wonder how long this could go on.

I contacted Connie again and asked her to update her brothers, especially about the morning meeting with the doctors. I wanted them to know about their mother's condition and the meeting so they could decide about coming to the hospital.

6-19-08

Here's the summary report from our house about how things have been going for the past few days. Sheila's condition is stable, Ernie the cat is clearly unstable, Hildey the dog is lonely, and I am glad that I've not met any more precocious children who are dog training experts. For important details, read on.

Sheila remains at OSU Hospital in the James Cancer facility. She is receiving very attentive and expert care, for which we are profoundly grateful. She has clearly survived the sepsis crisis, as all of her vital signs and blood tests are now normal. But there are two concerns to which the doctors are attending. One is the fact that the PICC line turned out to be the source of her infection. Since it was the means by which I hooked her up to the IV for her daily nutrition, there is a need for Plan B for feeding Sheila, whose digestive system continues to reject food. The pink tubs have been replaced by "beakers." Seems strange to me, but those beakers are what the staff wants her to use. The better to measure "output," I suppose. And, unfortunately, she is producing output on a daily basis.

The second concern is Sheila's bladder function. This is a new issue. Since her admission to the hospital, Sheila's urine has been very bloody. The doctors thought this would clear up. When it did not, they did a scope test (Sheila commented, "I've never seen the inside of my bladder before") to see what was going on and determined that the lining of her bladder is "inflamed" from her previous radiation treatments. In some cases, this clears up on its own, but in Sheila's case, the doctors recommended treatments in a hyperbolic chamber, the first of which occurred today. (Isn't this entire saga great for learning new things about medicine? We've had PICC lines and TPN, G-Tubes, gastric balloons, J-Tubes, Saline Flushes, Foleys, and now a hyperbolic chamber! Classic Sheila. She does not do things in moderation.)

Through all of this, Sheila is busy being Sheila. She really wants to get out of there and come home. In the meantime, she's learning the life history of everyone who tends to her (I could recite a litany you would not believe), and describing everything to me in some detail, including the location of her scope test and the hyperbolic chamber treatment as "the dungeon." "That room where they took me for the scope was a medieval torture chamber. The walls were lined with cabinets full of hoses and clamps and things you don't want to think about." And, of course, she did not appreciate her ride there in the hospital bed. She is adamant that hospitals need "ramps to get into the elevators." Have you looked at the floor when entering an elevator?! For my money, there is no place for a ramp. But Sheila continues to lobby for them anyway. Good luck.

My favorite interaction occurred the other evening when a young lady appeared at her door, was invited in (Sheila practices radical hospitality even when confined to a hospital bed), and this person said, "Hi, I'm Kerry, the Wednesday evening volunteer. Would you like a book or a magazine? We have lots of choices." Sheila instantly launched into her small talk on the way to learning this one's life story. I assessed her as the sort who does things well, is probably a candidate for an Ivy-league degree, and generally gives me hope for the next generation.

Nevertheless, Sheila concluded her small talk, listened to Kerry's recitation of the magazines she had, and said she wanted to read Money magazine. I nearly fell out of the chair. A woman who hasn't balanced her checkbook in years, pays professional people to help her manage her money, declines my offer to provide reading material every day, tells this kid she wants to read a Money magazine! I immediately began to speculate that "chemo brain" was impacting her more than I had realized. But I did not say anything.

Later in the evening when I was organizing the various things on the ever-present hospital tray, Sheila saw that magazine and said, "You can do whatever you want with that magazine. I won't read it. I took it because I didn't want to hurt that nice young girl's feelings." Forget chemo brain. Cancer and its treatments cannot destroy the essence of someone. I submit this story as evidence and rest my case.

Sheila continues to request no visitors. But please continue to send cards and pray for her. Sheila looks forward to my arrival with greetings from all of you and spends lots of time visiting with you via your cards. It's wonderful to observe and I thank you for making it possible for me to see.

More when I know more.

When I got to the hospital on Sunday, Sheila was sitting up in bed looking relatively well. But I was barely in the chair when she looked right at me and said, "The doctor was here today. He is a colleague of Dr. Cohn's. There is nothing more they can do for me. I want to go into hospice care now. At home. Please take me home." Her face had a pleading, but not pitiful look on it.

I took a moment to absorb what she was saying, recalled the image of her being all alone in that sterile ER room, and said, "I promise I will take you home." I meant that as much as I have meant anything I've ever said to another person.

I was not completely surprised. Dr. Cohn hinted at few options when he was in to see Sheila on Saturday morning and I assumed that subsequent testing and analysis confirmed that there were no more options. But hearing the news for sure was still a jolt. Sheila had fought through a seriously compromised quality of life for six months, and it was time to acknowledge that it was time to let go.

We just sat there together for a short while, not saying anything. "I wanted to tell you first," she finally said. "Now I have to call the kids and grandkids. Can you bring me their phone numbers? The people here are making an appointment with the hospice people, so there are some things to work out. I want Mt. Carmel Hospice. I know about their good work from when Allan was sick. They said it's ok if I use Mt. Carmel instead of OSU."

I was shifting into extremely high look-out-for-Sheila mode. In my private thoughts at that moment, I resolved to help her through the end of her life by doing whatever she needed, as directed by Sheila herself or her hospice nurses. Nobody and nothing else would matter. I focused first on getting her home and resolved to do anything necessary to get her out of there as soon as possible.

We located Connie's phone number and Sheila called her to tell her what was going on. Connie provided all other phone numbers and I sat with Sheila while she called her sons. She had shifted into "look-out-for-everyone-else" mode, so was delivering her news with a reassuring tone that she was at peace with her decision and had full confidence in the hospice people. It was an impressive display of faith, consideration for others, and decisiveness, all hallmarks of Sheila throughout her life.

Later that day, the doctor who had been treating her in Dr. Cohn's absence came in to see her. He briefly reviewed her medical status, the fact that no additional treatments were recommended, and that she agreed to be discharged in the care of hospice.

This tall robust doctor then crouched down at the bedside of his failing patient, took her hand and said, "I'm very sorry we can't do anything else for you, Mrs. Zinn. It has been my honor to know you briefly and to treat you these past few days. I hope things go well for you when you get home. If you have any questions or concerns, please call us. I think you will be in excellent hands with the hospice service."

I had never seen a doctor say goodbye to a patient before. I hope everybody's doctor does as well as that man did that day. He shook my hand on the way out and expressed his sorrow to me about not being able to do more. Yes, I was sorry too. But I was sure that these skilled and conscientious doctors had done everything possible. This was a reassuring thought to have in the face of this harsh reality

As I got up to leave her several hours later, Sheila looked at me again and said, "Please take me home." I again assured her that I would take her home, even if we had to do a midnight escape out the back door. That made her laugh. But I was deadly serious.

On Monday, I went to the office. Sheila was still waiting for discharge orders and confirmation from the Mt. Carmel hospice people that they were ready to implement her intake processes. The plan was for her to call me to confirm what time to pick her up.

I didn't hear from her until midafternoon when she said I could come any time. When I got to the hospital, her daughter-in-law Tina (Mark's wife and a very capable person) was there. I was very glad for her presence. She was helping Sheila organize her few belongings and was talking very positively about Sheila going home.

Soon it was time for me to get the car to meet them in the front of the hospital. I took off to navigate through the hospital complex to the parking garage. On the way, it occurred to me that I wasn't sure I could get Sheila into the house by myself. The step into the house from the garage was out. The Cokes and bricks were long gone and I didn't have time to reconstruct them. Access via the front sidewalk required no steps at all, but would require a longer walk that I wasn't sure Sheila could do. I knew I couldn't hold her up the entire way. I had visions of her collapsing in a heap on our front sidewalk.

I called Tina's cell phone as I walked, explained my concerns, and asked her to meet me at the house. She understood the need and assured me she would be there to assist in getting Sheila into the house. The hospital people helped me get Sheila into the car and we took off. As we were driving home, Tina called my cell phone. She was stuck in the OSU parking garage (what *IS* it with that place and the parking?!) because she was trying to leave just when many hospital workers were ending their shifts. She would not beat me home, as we originally planned. But, bless Tina, she called Connie, who lived five minutes from our house and arranged for Connie to meet us in the driveway. Connie was there.

Sheila was home.

6-24-08

Friends, this is the one e-mail that I did not want to write nor do you want to read. But I now have to tell you that, after extensive consultation with her doctors about the lack of progress in treating her condition, Sheila has decided to discontinue treatment and come home from the hospital under the care of the Mt. Carmel Hospice professionals. She made this decision over the weekend while still in the hospital and took some time to notify her children and brother before asking me to communicate with all of you.

We came home last evening relatively uneventfully, laden with various items from the hospital that the nurses wanted us to have (tape, gauze dressings, lotions, more pink tubs) and Sheila settled into her favorite chair in the family room.

The hospice intake nurse arrived for a meeting with the family around 8:00 p.m. She reviewed the services provided by them and answered any and all questions. I think we are all very comfortable that we will receive excellent support from them as things unfold.

Sheila, despite being very tired, made everyone laugh when she responded to a question from the nurse about her height and weight. She said, "Well, over the years, I've been growing wider and shrinking in height so I look like Sponge Bob Square Pants." And, true to form, she lied about her weight because she has no idea what she weighs. It's been an inside joke with us caregivers because someone has been calling every week inquiring about her weight and Sheila makes something up every week!

Additional news that you should understand is that the doctors told Sheila yesterday that she is also experiencing kidney failure. This will cause events to unfold "more quickly" than otherwise would be so, but timelines are not discussed so I have nothing to relay to you along those lines.

Today, the nurse who will be in charge of Sheila's case was here for a very long time. His name is Tom and she likes him very much. He's thorough, compassionate, and exudes confidence about handling anything and everything. He already has several things in motion to make Sheila more safe and comfortable here at home. Fortunately, she is experiencing no pain and is mostly comfortable other than the nausea and we're working on that.

Connie, Mark, and I are continuing our routine of providing daily care for Sheila and I'm also here evenings, nights, and weekends. In addition, other family members are providing much needed moral and practical support. Sheila's brother is planning to come for a visit sometime in the next several days and she is looking forward to that.

I don't know how to close this note other than to again thank all of you for your support and to ask that you continue to send cards and pray for Sheila. Please don't stop now. Those efforts are very sustaining. I will provide additional updates when I can. And we will see this through in a fashion that is true to Sheila's wishes.

The meeting with the hospice intake nurse made me crazy. There were eleven people (three kids and spouses, granddaughter and spouse, nurse, Sheila, me) packed into our family room, sitting in a large circle. Sheila was in her chair beside the nurse. I understand that they have processes to follow, but the questioning and endless paperwork was really trying my patience. The presence of this audience for such a process was making me anxious. I wanted Sheila to myself at our home for a moment. I wanted to have quiet time with her and time to talk with her about what was coming.

I tried to understand Sheila's desire to have everyone there. "They need to understand that I am fine with this choice and they need to be involved to hear again how hospice works."

The intake nurse was doing full disclosure on how everything would work. She had Sheila publicly state her intentions, and asked who the primary caregiver would be. I didn't say anything, but waited to see if one of the kids wanted to claim that. I would have deferred to them, had they wanted to handle things that way. And I was watching Sheila. She caught my eye and gave me a look that told me to speak in the face of the brief silence that filled the room. "I am the primary caregiver," I said.

The house was very busy during the week. Connie and Mark came on their scheduled days. Steve arrived, and Allan had become more involved. I talked to Sheila one evening about my schedule and we agreed that I would keep going to the office, since people were around to keep her company during the day.

In my mind, I was trying to figure out how to manage my time off. All family members of people in hospice care must go through this. If you start vacation time too soon, you may run out of it or be absent from work responsibilities longer than is manageable. If you wait too long, you may be deprived of precious time with your loved one at the end of life. There is no magic timetable, I learned. So I decided to take my cues from the hospice nurses and Sheila who said, "I am very well-tended-to here. I want to make some phone calls to my aunts and to Joe (her grandson in Alabama), so you should go."

I needed some time in the office to get back-up people organized to handle things when I would be out. I also wanted to talk to my boss about her expectations. So I was in the office, working shorter days than usual, but I went in each day.

I have a hard time remembering what happened that week, other than several distinct things. One was Sheila talking to me about wanting to invite the pastor over to plan her funeral. I offered to make the call for her, but she clearly intended to handle it herself. She did and on Thursday, Pastor Ruth came while I was at the office and Mark was at the house. They planned Sheila's funeral.

Sheila talked to me about her preferences in general when I got home and asked how their meeting had gone. But she did not offer too many specifics other than she hoped the choir could sing and "maybe the handbells could ring, but people are very busy, so

I wouldn't want to inconvenience anyone. The directors will have to see who's available." Yes, I would have expected that kind of a thought from her. I told her I was pretty sure that members of both groups—especially the handbell choir which Sheila had directed for ten years—would do everything possible to be available for her service if they knew that's what she wanted.

The other thing I remember so clearly is talking to Sheila about her obituary. I knew this was a big deal to her. Early in the week, I suggested that she work on it so it would be just how she wanted it to be. She agreed to spend time on it. Nothing happened.

The next day, I suggested that she at least make a list of things she wanted to include, since there were major parts of her life that I knew nothing about and that her kids might not know, either. Yes, she would do that. Nothing happened.

Finally, toward the end of the week when we had a brief private moment, I asked her if she wanted me to draft her obituary. She looked right into my eyes and said, "Yes, I think I will need a little help with that. I would appreciate it."

Later that evening when someone was visiting with her, I went upstairs to our office and sat down at the same computer I had been using for months to update her friends and family about her condition and I wrote Sheila's obituary for her. We had never really talked about how she wanted it to be, even after all her comments about writing it herself so it would be just the way she wanted. I felt inadequate, but I wanted to get something down so she could see it. I wanted her to read it and talk to me so I could change it to be just how she wanted it. It was clear that she could not do it alone. I wanted to help her with it.

I tried to remember everything she had accomplished. As I struggled to write, I remember thinking that I had never done anything quite so bizarre. I was sitting in the office of my own home writing the obituary of my closest friend who was downstairs visiting with extended family members, probably for the final time. I hated it. I didn't want to be doing it. I had to read the words I was typing and I didn't want to acknowledge the impending reality of them. But I kept going. Something compelled me to keep going.

When I finished, I printed it out and went downstairs to show it to Sheila, whose only company then was Connie and Tina. "See what you think of this," I said and handed the paper to her.

She read it very carefully and then looked up and said, "It's just right. Please add that I died 'after a courageous battle with cancer.' Thank you for doing that," and handed the paper to Connie. Connie became preoccupied by the location of a comma, which was debated with her mother for a short while. Nothing was decided and Sheila kept the paper beside her chair. "I want to show it to Mark and Allan when they come by again."

During the next several days, I asked Sheila if she wanted me to change anything in her obituary. "No, I like it just the way it is." To this day, I wonder if she was just being polite or if I had really accomplished what she had long envisioned. I suspect the former, unfortunately.

Another thing I remember from that week is that Sheila began to talk about her possessions. We had wording in the legal trust agreement which stated that the survivor would be responsible to distribute family possessions to the deceased's family. The attorneys had encouraged us to enumerate our respective possessions, but we rejected that suggestion. We knew which things were precious to the other family and trusted each other to handle the distribution at the right time. The trust also stated that the distribution would only happen when the survivor authorized it.

Sheila only ever talked to me about three possessions: her piano, a ring, and the dog. "I want Claire (her granddaughter, a music major in college) and Tony (her husband, also a music major) to have the piano. But they have that little tiny house and won't have room for it. I think you're going to have to sell the piano."

"Sheila, I think they will be honored and thrilled to have that piano They will find a way to fit it into their home, I'll bet." I thought this was the end of the discussion. I was wrong.

Several days later; "I think you're going to have to sell the piano. Claire and Tony won't have room for it. I would love for them to have it, but we have to be realistic."

"Sheila, I will never sell your piano. Never. Someone else might at some point. But I will never do that. If Claire and Tony don't have room for the piano, I will keep it here until they do."

"But you might move and not have room for it."

"I might, but I will not sell it. I will pay for it to be in a climate-controlled storage building until they can take it."

"That would be very expensive."

"I can afford it. If something happens and I cannot afford it anymore and they still are not ready to take it, I will go get another job before I sell that piano. I am very serious, Sheila. I will never sell your piano. Claire, Tony, and I will work something out. I think they will be thrilled to have it and I will be sure they get it." She studied my "I mean it" face for a few moments and said nothing. We didn't talk about the piano being sold again.

She also mentioned a ring that meant a lot to her. It was gold with an aqua-colored stone in it. The aqua was her favorite color and she was so pleased with the ring when it was made for her. She wore it constantly before her hospitalization. She wanted me to have it. I wear it often now myself, especially when I'm remembering something that makes me feel close to her.

Sheila also talked to me about Hildey one evening when just the two of us and the dog were sitting in the family room. Hildey looked up attentively when Sheila shifted her position in the chair. "Awww.... Isn't she cute? You will look after her when I'm gone, won't you?"

I replied, "Sheila, I promise I will do right by your dog."

6-28-08

Well, we've had an interesting week. Sheila has become weaker and sicker. The rest of us are becoming sadder as we face the reality of the unfolding events, but we remain committed to providing the best experiences and home environment possible for Sheila during her final weeks with us.

We have felt very much supported by the Mt. Carmel Hospice team. Sheila's case manager nurse, Tom, is very compassionate, responsive, and easy to deal with. So are the on-call nurses. Sheila also received the services of a home health aide for bathing this past week, and received a visit from a social worker sort who will assist with paperwork and other administrative activities.

I would say that things have become more uncomfortable for Sheila as the week has progressed. We successfully avoided use of the pink tub for almost five days, but the need for it has returned within the past 24 hours, and all too frequently. I am working with the nurses to make adjustments to medications so we can hopefully get the nausea under control.

Sheila and I had an eventful night on Wednesday when the storms rolled through. She was restless as she went to bed that evening (she is still moving from her bed in the dining room to her chair in the family room and back on a daily basis) so I sat with her and talked or just held her hand. I value this time very much because it's when she talks to me about what's on her mind ("I think all of the kids and grandkids will be OK" or she tells me "Ma Thaxton was right. It's hard to get into this world and hard to get out" or "I just want to go see Jesus") and I reassure her that she's doing fine with everything.

She had just become settled and I had gone up to my room to bed and turned on the monitor I use to listen for her, when a very shrill sound jolted me out of the initial phases of what I had hoped would be peaceful sleep. I sat bolt upright in my bed, slightly disoriented for a moment, and then realized that Sheila's weather radio alarm was sounding downstairs in her bedroom. I cursed that thing yet again because I have not liked it since she got it. But it makes her feel secure, so I had moved it down there for her.

I flew out of bed, raced down the hall, took the steps as fast as I could, tripped over the throw rug at the bottom of the steps, got tangled up in the curtain that separates her room from the hallway, and slammed into a box of medical supplies on my way to that despicable alarm. I had determined that, in the moment that it took me to recognize what had caused the disruption of Sheila's rest, that the alarm was now mine to control and it was about to be a goner. I yanked the plug from the wall, remembered the battery back-up from a previous run-in with this device, turned it over, opened every door on the back of the thing until I found a battery, jerked the battery from the plastic connection, and dropped that whole mess into the box of medical supplies feeling very triumphant.

Sheila, of course, could hardly miss my arrival and began to express her concerns about the weather. She wanted me to "go get the dog" (she must be kidding) and usher everyone to the basement so we didn't get blown away by the tornado she was sure was on the way. This moment obviously called for some of my persuasive abilities and I began my "sale" of there being no imminent danger. "It's just a thunderstorm warning," I told her. I no sooner got those words out of my mouth and she began to settle down when the Franklin County tornado warning siren located across the road from us went off. I could not believe it. I immediately told Sheila that we needed to see the TV for an update.

I raced back up the steps to an upstairs TV so she would not get too invested in all of this, and saw that the problem was in Hilliard and headed for Bexley. Good news! (sorry to those of you who live in either community). I hauled back down the steps and told Sheila that we had no problem in Grove City and I would keep watching the TV, which I did.

All was well with that and around 1:00 a.m. everyone, including the dog, settled down, until 3:00 a.m. when the baby monitor began beeping a malfunction alarm that awakened me. I determined that the problem was not on my end. So it was back out of bed, down the steps, across the rug, through the curtain, and into Sheila's room where her end of the monitor resides. This time, I went slowly and quietly because there was no way for her to know anything was up. I fumbled with the thing as quietly as possible, did nothing more profound than unplugging and re-plugging and said "thank you" to the blasted thing when it turned green again. I tell you, a person knows they're getting weary when inanimate objects become worthy of thanks.

As for the important events of the week, Sheila has been able to enjoy visits from her children and grandchildren this week. Her brother arrived on Thursday evening and will be here through the weekend. He wanted to time his visit to be here when she could converse with him and they've been able to do that. So I think he made a decision that was good for both of them.

Sheila is so appreciative of the many cards she is receiving. They enable me to distract her from her discomfort for a short while. She reads each one carefully and comments on how nice everyone is to take time to write to her. It is very touching to see her receive back from all of you what I know she's given to you within your friendships. And thanks to those who write to me, too. It is very important to me to do this well and I'm working very hard at it in honor of my friend.

I told Sheila earlier today that I was going to send an update and invited her to recommend something for me to include. She said, "Tell them I don't know if I'll really miss them all that much because where I'll be, everything will be better." She always makes me laugh, even now!

Thanks for your support. Time to get the patient to bed!

We began to have some rough nights as the week went on. Sheila was restless at night, sometimes in pain, and I decided that the baby monitor arrangement was insufficient. I located an inflatable mattress that we had folded up in the closet from the last time my family visited, and I inflated it. "I'm going to put this in the floor right beside your bed, so I'm closer to you at night," I explained to her. I received no resistance to this plan and didn't plan to listen if I had.

Sheila was still getting out of bed every day and moving to her chair in the family room. Her declaration, "I've seen hospice patients resist getting into bed for the last time. It must be awful to know that you're not getting up again. I'm the same way. I can understand it better now."

I was not resting very well. Sheila's restlessness and my preoccupation with providing top notch care just did not allow me to relax very effectively. The hospice nurses were absolutely wonderful at responding to Sheila's needs when they were at the house in the evenings and I described her condition. They made adjustments to the medications I administered, talked to her and listened carefully when she described how she was feeling. I was greatly reassured by their presence, even if by phone.

After I wrote the last update to the e-mail crowd, I realized that at some point, I would be telling them that Sheila had died. I wanted to do that with some sensitivity and in a way that properly honored our friend. So one evening, bizarreness returned in our office, as I drafted my final note to the email group. I wasn't sure I would be in a condition to communicate effectively after Sheila died, so I wrote the announcement of her death while she was sitting downstairs with her brother.

Mark knew that the nights were rough for me because Sheila told him about our escapades beyond the weather (pain meds, mild sedatives). He offered to come and stay one night so I could catch up on rest. I thanked him and deferred, telling him that I was planning to start taking days off the following week. "Let's see how the weekend goes," I said.

By Saturday, I was really feeling lousy. I did my best to hide it from Sheila and asked Mark if he could stay on Monday night. I knew he had to work on Sunday. We made plans for him to take night duty on Monday.

Saturday night was not relaxing for Sheila or me. She just could not get comfortable in her bed, had a hard time describing how she was feeling, and the medications that the nurse suggested by phone did not seem to help as much as we all would have liked. During one of the very early morning calls, the hospice nurse said, "We're not making progress. She should not be so uncomfortable. We're going to send someone out to the house to see her tomorrow. You both need things to be better."

I immediately felt a release of the tension that had been building as I tried my best to administer to Sheila, but could see that she was not comfortable. I was amazed that the night-duty hospice nurse always answered the phone, sounding like she had nothing better to do than listen to and advise me. And now she was using her professional judgment and experience to diagnose that we needed help. She communicated gently and reassuringly. Her "take charge and do something" attitude delivered just what I needed, mostly because I wanted expert care for Sheila and I was not providing it. This skilled physical and emotional care that we received is the reason that I continue to support the work of hospice organizations, especially Mt. Carmel in Columbus, Ohio.

Sheila got up as usual and moved to her chair on Sunday morning. I explained that a hospice nurse was coming to see us in the afternoon (they called to confirm the time). Steve was at the house to be with her, I was going to church, and taking the dog to the groomer on the way (not ordinarily a good idea to get in a car with an excited dog on a Sunday morning, but these circumstances were extraordinary. She needed it. It was the best I could do).

When I got home with the dog, Sheila was in her chair, feeling "fine" and Steve went out for a bit. Sheila and Hildey did their dog greeting thing and then everybody settled down. It was the first time since we had started this journey with hospice that we had some time during the day to talk. I knelt beside her chair and asked her if she wanted anything. "No, I'm doing okay, considering."

I smiled at her and said, "I'm really going to miss you. I don't know how I'll manage without you." Tears filled my eyes and trickled down my cheeks, the first tears I shed in Sheila's presence since this whole thing began in January. She wiped them from my face gently and said, "You'll be fine. You're strong. I'm not worried about you."

I tried to smile again and then said something that she had taught me is vital to say to a loved one who is dying, "Sheila, I hope you know that it's fine for you to go. I want to say it to you again. When it is time for you to go see God, you go. You go when you are ready." She nodded and I stood up because the doorbell rang. The hospice nurse had arrived.

Joann was perfect. She assessed Sheila's condition, listened to her, and listened to me. She told me she thought Sheila needed a catheter and some changes in her medications so she could be more comfortable. She knelt by Sheila's chair, just where I had been moments prior, took her hand, and explained the plan. I had warned her that Sheila sometimes had plans of her own and might resist.

The woman had the perfect touch and I helped Sheila move to the bed and then left while Joann worked to get Sheila more comfortable. In a short while, Joann moved into the kitchen and I joined her from the family room. "She's settled now. I think this will be better. Be sure to call us if that changes. You have our number, don't you?"

"Are you kidding? I've called that number at least three times in the middle of the night for the past two nights. I have it committed to memory," I thought and almost smiled. I assured her that I would call if I needed help and thanked her for coming to help us. She assured me that she had reviewed all the file notes and that my late night calls were appropriate and that her presence today was a good decision by her colleague. I felt like a validated care-giver. Another great gift I received during this time.

Before she left, I wanted her to help me estimate how much longer Sheila would live. She was quite non-committal but in the process of checking on my supply of meds, she thought I needed more than the three-day supply I already had.

I decided that with Friday of the next week being the Fourth of July holiday, I would work another two days and then start taking extended time off to be home with Sheila. Steve was going back to Alabama on Monday morning. Sheila's children and I could usher her through this. I envisioned periods of her being in and out of awareness over several days as her body slowly shut down.

Joann left and Steve came back, settling into the family room to watch TV. Sheila was sleeping deeply and seemed comfortable, something I attributed to Joann's ministrations. I didn't want to watch Fox News that Steve had on, nobody else was around, I couldn't settle down to read, so I just sat with Sheila, watching her rest. Sometimes I moved into the living room and sat there. I really did not know what to do with myself. I didn't want to leave her, but she didn't need anything, either. Time seemed to be suspended.

Sheila rallied a bit in the early evening and talked to me about feeling pain. I got her some pain medications and we talked about little things for a while until she relaxed again. It was looking like it would be a restful night. I was glad Sheila could get some rest after two prior nights of too little sleep for both of us.

Steve went to bed and I organized my mattress on the floor. We all settled down earlier than usual. I heard Sheila awaken once, got her settled, and heard her again when she wanted pain medication around midnight. I easily tended to her. But she complained again in a short while and it was too soon to administer more meds. My instructions were to call the hospice nurse on call. I got Beth. She told me what to do and implored me to call her back in an hour so she could hear me describe Sheila's response to the meds I had given her. I talked to Beth at 1:00 a.m. and reported that Sheila was not completely settled, but seemed better. "Wait another half an hour and call me again," she suggested. "We want to be sure she has a good night. There are more things we can do if she's still not comfortable. Please call me."

I called her. This time, Sheila was quite settled. I assured Beth that I would hear Sheila if she needed me again. And I would call Beth if I was uncertain what to do. I couldn't believe I slept for three hours and heard nothing. I had a clock on the floor and woke up startled to see that it was just after 6:00 a.m.

I sat up and peeked over the side of the bed to look at Sheila. She was completely still in an awkward position on the bed. I touched her gently, trying to rouse her. No response. I was on my knees now, nudging her more urgently. No response.

"No, this cannot be. She can't be gone. I cannot have slept through it. I was going to call the kids to come. Nobody was with her. I was sleeping on the floor. She cannot be gone."

I jumped up and pulled on a shirt over the night shirt and sweat pants I had slept in. "No." I kept thinking. "No, it's not supposed to be like this. We never really had time to say goodbye. Her children aren't here. Everybody missed it. This just can't be. I wanted to be with her, holding her hand. I wanted her to know I was with her when she died. This cannot be."

I walked from the dining room to the kitchen and leaned on the counter, trying to think, trying to jolt myself out of sleep. I kept thinking about her children and having to tell them that their mother died and I didn't call them. "It's too soon," I kept thinking. "We needed more time."

Finally I realized that I couldn't just keep standing there insisting that reality wasn't real just because I didn't want it to be. I called Beth. "My patient died. I think my patient died," I said quietly into the phone. Then she gave me the great gift of a thought to hold on to, "Many people die the way they live." I realized then that in Sheila's case, it was in not wanting to inconvenience anybody.

"We will send someone right over," Beth said. "Are you alone?"

"Yes, but I won't be for long."

Mark would be coming through the door very shortly expecting to stay with his mother for the day while I went to the office for a while. Connie and Dave would be going out the door to work very shortly. Allan and Kay had to be notified. I had to get with it.

I called Connie's house and Dave answered. I told him what happened. "We'll be right over."

As I was hanging up the phone, Mark came through the door and I told him, "I'm sorry, Mark. It's too soon. The hospice people ordered more medicine. I expected at least another week."

"It's okay. Nobody can predict these things. I have to call Tina. Would you like me to call Allan, too?"

"Yes. Thank you." I sat at the kitchen table, then in my sweatpants and flannel shirt with my long hair tumbling all over the place, and I waited for the hospice person and Sheila's other children to come. I did not shed a tear. I just sat there.

To their enduring credit, none of them expressed disappointment or anger to me at having not been present for their mother's death. They went about the necessary business with a cooperative spirit and worked well together.

Once the family members were all there and Sheila's body had been moved, they began their plans for visiting the funeral home later in the day. I offered to call the pastor and did so at their request. Connie and Tina went to Sheila's closet and began discussions about what clothes to take to the funeral home. I did not care about that and did not participate.

They invited me to go with them to the funeral home, but I declined. I had done the bulk of the care-giving. I gave myself permission to opt out of funeral home discussions, especially because Sheila had never expressed any opinions on any of that. I felt like I didn't have to advocate for her in that arena. Whatever they wanted and decided would be fine.

I was surprised when Tina called from the funeral home that afternoon. "Nancy, we're reviewing this obituary you wrote for final approval. We noticed that you didn't put yourself in it.

We think you should be mentioned. Did you leave yourself out intentionally?"

I was stunned that they had thought of it. I honestly had not. I just wrote the classic obituary with blood relatives listed as survivors. Sheila and I never talked about that and she never said anything when she reviewed my version. That's what I told Tina. I thanked her for thinking about including me and told her that whatever they decided was fine. They put me in. I was touched.

I waited until later in the day to write to the e-mail friends. I wanted to include information on the arrangements, so I could write one last note to that group. I re-read what I had drafted and kept it mostly as I had written it, glad I had composed it in advance. As I sat to write the last e-mail, I realized that I would miss my correspondent friends. It had been therapeutic somehow for me to write to them. These dear and devoted friends of Sheila's had shared the journey with me. I was going to miss them and I felt our shared pain of her death excruciatingly.

6-30-08

I am very sad to tell you that Sheila died early this morning. This was a bit sooner than everyone, including our hospice experts, anticipated. But everyone is glad that she is not sick any more.

Sheila had a pretty uncomfortable weekend and the hospice people sent someone out yesterday afternoon to assess her. The nurse, Joann, was terrific and tended to Sheila with strength and warmth and a very strong desire to make her more comfortable. She outlined a new regimen of medicine, ordered refills for supplies beyond the several days' supply we had on hand, and predicted nothing in terms of a timeline when I asked.

I gave Sheila medicine at midnight according to the new plan and she was beginning to rest more peacefully. She was due for additional medicines at 4 a.m. and I was quite confident I would hear her stirring about so I could administer that dose. It was not to be.

I slept until 6:15 this morning and soon thereafter determined that Sheila had passed on during the night. When I called the hospice people, the nurse on call (to whom I had spoken many times in the wee hours of recent nights) said, "Wow; that was fast. And you should know that some of our patients do die when nobody is around because they don't want to trouble anyone by making them maintain a vigil or watch them struggle a bit. They just want to go when it will cause the least trouble for everyone. Was your friend like that?" Yes, that's our Sheila!

Sheila's children have been here all day and are working together to complete arrangements for their mother. There was even some levity as they recalled many great moments from her life, despite the profound loss they are feeling.

Calling hours for Sheila will be on Wednesday from 2–4 p.m. and 6–8 p.m. at the church. The funeral service will be at 10 a.m. on Thursday at the church. The church is Trinity United Methodist Church, 4850 Haughn Road, Grove City, Ohio. In lieu of flowers, Sheila requested donations to either Heifer International or Mt. Carmel Hospice.

As for me, I hardly know how to express what is in my heart and mind now. Sheila and I lived together for 12 years. And they were great years. We traveled all over the world, had parties with friends, hosted countless family visits and birthday parties, and just plain enjoyed each other's company.

I loved Sheila's musicianship, sense of humor, determination, commitment to fighting things that she deemed "unfair," her high-spiritedness, her love of family, and her faith. I will miss those things beyond what I can imagine now.

Sheila made this household a home that communicated a warm welcome to all, made radical hospitality a reality, and provided the "breakfast" part of "bed and breakfast" (sorry, folks but we're only "bed" now).

Sheila taught me many things about the arts, resourcefulness, and patience. Beyond all things, she modeled kindness. She told me one time that she thought her life would be a good one if the words on her tombstone could truthfully say "She was kind." I think she passed with flying colors. She was kind to all people and all of God's creatures. If she was unkind occasionally, it was to herself.

After Allan died, Sheila told me that she didn't want to remember him as a sick person, but she wanted to remember him for all the other things that defined him. I now understand how she felt. Sheila's presence in my life was an incredible gift to me. I am heartbroken by her absence but forever enriched by her eternal presence.

The next several days are hard to remember. Several things do stick in my mind from that time. I remember becoming obsessive about getting the empty hospital bed out of the dining room. The hospice people made all the arrangements and assured me that it would be picked up on Tuesday. I couldn't stand to even look in the dining room where Sheila and I had spent so many hours together during the final months of her life. The empty bed was just too much.

The supply people came for the IV pole and pump early in the day. I was glad to see them go. When the bed was still there early afternoon, I decided that it had to be gone by the end of the day and I was going to make sure it was. I think I called the hospice office first and they provided the number of the supply company. Once I located the proper people in that office, they assured me that their driver was scheduled for a stop at our house and would be there by the end of the day. Despite their assurances, I was still on edge about getting that bed out of the house.

There were some other distractions that day, thankfully. I asked a friend to come by to help me arrange food for the time between two sessions of calling hours. Pastor Ruth stopped by and confirmed that the church people were handling a meal after the funeral service. The kids came by to look through photos for the display at calling hours. And late in the afternoon, the company came to pick up the hospital bed. The knot of tension in my stomach that I had been living with for months was loosened just a tad at that departure.

The next day I remember that I didn't want to do it, but the house was quiet and I had some time, so I ventured into the dining room to work on removing the other things that had accumulated in there, so it could return to being the dining room again. I folded up the throw rugs, took the curtain rod down, got rid of the boxes of medical supplies that the hospice people couldn't re-deploy, and reached for the Rubbermaid stacking drawers.

My energy was waning from the task of getting the room back in order when I pulled open the top drawer and the first thing I saw was Sheila's purple underwear. That underwear had been a joke for some time. I had been headed out to Kohl's one evening about a year prior to use a gift card and take advantage of a sale. I was going to buy underwear for myself. Sheila wanted me to get some for her too and provided specific instructions on size and "make sure the underpants are interesting."

"Sheila, how in the world does anyone make underwear interesting? I'm going to Kohl's, not Victoria's Secret."

"I mean colorful. Don't just get white or off-white."

I came home with purple and she loved it. Every time we did laundry, I would make a comment about her "interesting" underwear.

I dissolved into tears when I opened that drawer and saw her purple underwear. I sat on my little stool there and just cried for a while. No more underwear jokes on laundry day. No more jokes ever with Sheila again. These were my first tears since she had died and they were tears of pain and emptiness.

Then, it occurred to me that if she were around we would have a good laugh about me sitting in our dining room crying over her purple underwear. I stood up, collected all the underwear from the drawer, and threw it in the trash. And I cleaned out the other contents of those drawers and took the empty drawers to the basement. I didn't want to see them for a while. After a few hours, the dining room was ready to be a dining room again.

I remember that Steve had to go out and buy some dress clothes. He had expected to return to Alabama after his visit with Sheila and before her death, so he now had to make new arrangements.

I remember Margie calling to confirm that the bells would ring and to get my "approval" of the piece she had in mind.

I remember being surprised at how many of my colleagues came to the calling hours and how many of Sheila's friends—some of whom I had never met thanked me profusely for the e-mail correspondence. In many cases they drew me into tight, warm embraces sharing the pain of our loss.

I remember that my brother and his family drove seven hours from Pennsylvania to attend the calling hours and the funeral. When they had done what they could for me at the church, I encouraged them to go to the house and wait for me. As they left, they asked what they might do to help and when I got home I found my dining room had been re-established.

And, I remember that despite its being vibrant aqua, I decided to wear my blazer of Sheila's favorite color to her funeral.

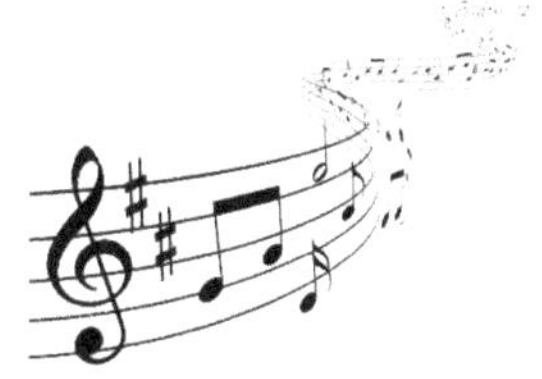

Full Measure

7-5-08

After these many months of correspondence with you about Sheila's health, I want to write a few more words before signing off as your communication liaison.

Foremost, thank you for your support for Sheila in cards and prayers. Many people expressed a desire to help during Sheila's illness and it was true that what she wanted and needed was for you to pray for her and write to her. You all came through with flying colors! I tried to convey how much it meant to Sheila that you maintained your prayer and mail vigilance and I'm saying again how much it meant to her to receive these things from her cherished friends.

I also want to tell you how affirming it was for me to meet many of you during the services for Sheila this past week. It's always good to place names and faces together and I'm glad that so many of you introduced yourselves to me. I also appreciate your kind expressions of gratitude for my correspondence over these many months. I am very glad that you felt informed about Sheila's condition and connected to her through the e-mails. And I'm thankful for the many expressions of sympathy sent my way from all of you.

Many of you asked about my future plans. I plan to be here for a while, probably until I retire. The house feels very comfortable to me despite Sheila's absence from it and I don't plan to make any quick decisions to change big things. So you can reach me at the home address for the foreseeable future.

Now we all have to figure out how to carry on in the face of this profound loss. For me, that means remaining faithful in response to God's faithfulness through all of this (Sheila and I saw God's presence everywhere over these past few months), establishing new household routines, honoring my wonderful friend in appropriate ways at appropriate times, and figuring out how in the world to be a dog owner. I'm going to do the best I can taking one day at a time. I wish you all the best of everything and thank you again for your presence through the final months of Sheila's life.

I was glad when things calmed down after Sheila's funeral. Steve went back to Alabama, the house returned to pre-illness state, and I tried to get on with my new reality. In the process of doing that, I resolved to listen to my own advice; handling the grief process in my own way.

I spent hours writing thank you notes. Sheila was fanatic about writing thank you notes. I used to accuse her of writing thank you notes for thank you notes. I swear she did that at least once, although she always denied it. Diligence with thank you notes felt like a form of honoring her.

I had local people to thank for their many kindnesses and I had people to thank for making contributions in lieu of flowers. Sheila had requested donations to Heifer International and Mt. Carmel Hospice. Both organizations were relatively prompt at sending notifications to the house after contributions were made. The majority were neighbors, church friends, my friends, and Sheila's friends. If I didn't recognize names, the kids did.

Sheila died on June 30 and I was still writing thank you notes for contributions in August as notifications kept coming in. Once again, her friends were generous in tending to her wishes.

I also wrote letters to Dr. Chambers and Dr. Cohn, thanking them for their conscientious and expert care for Sheila. Those men were impressive professionals who worked diligently to cure Sheila, and in the absence of that, to make the quality of her life as good as it could be.

I remember that within four or five days after Sheila's funeral, my friend Lisa gently prodded me to think about a new routine for feeding myself. All during Sheila's hospitalization and illness at home, I had modified my approach to meals. I ate breakfast every day, but relied on the office cafeteria at noon time for any hot food. I only ate fruit or yogurt or crackers in the evenings when tending to Sheila. Since she could not eat and loved food, it seemed insensitive for me to do anything other than snacking.

Lisa helped me plan several casseroles, a grocery list, and scheduled a day while I was still on my five-day bereavement leave to come over and cook with me. We made the casseroles and divided them into single-serving containers for my freezer, an approach that had worked for me prior to life with Sheila. Lisa was relieved that I wouldn't starve and her kindness made me face the new reality of my life.

In early August I went to the beach with my brother's family for a week. It was nice to change scenery, although I'm not sure I was very good company. I had time to think about things I needed to do now that the thank-you notes were winding down. I had to think about the distribution of the family items in the house to the kids. I didn't want to wait too long out of respect for their mother's wishes and their own need to have the things. Connie was also talking about the need to sell Sheila's car since nobody in the family wanted it.

When I got home, I contacted the kids and invited them to the house. After we visited for a while, I reviewed the provisions of the trust with them even though they all had copies of it. I invited them to make preparations to take the family things out of the house whenever they were ready. We talked about which things would go, so there was no confusion, and they quickly decided who would take what, leaving some things to be determined later. They were very agreeable with each other and very nice to me.

What I was not ready for was the physical transformation of the house. I should have anticipated it, but I didn't. The emptiness of the dining room without the antique corner cupboard, picture hooks on the walls where paintings had hung, the rocking chair that had been Blanche's favorite no longer at the bottom of the steps, the kitchen cupboards with empty spaces where dishes once were stacked; parts of my house were a wreck. The place that we had made so comfortable and that had been so comforting became distressing to me.

This happened over a period of several months as precious family things were relocated. I was able to make the family room into a place of some sanctuary, but only after I made some changes. I called the local furniture bank and donated Sheila's chair to them. It was one of a matching pair that we had bought just a year or two prior. It pained me terribly to see that empty chair. I tried sitting in it, but felt like a wholly inadequate replacement for the person who usually occupied it. Thus the decision to give it away and rearrange the furniture. That helped, and I found a place to be comfortable in my house.

The piano was next. I waited until some of the initial big things had been removed, then contacted Claire and asked if she and Tony could come by sometime because I had something I wanted to give them from her grandmother.

When they arrived on a Sunday afternoon, we sat in the living room near the piano and I told them what Sheila wanted for her piano. I didn't tell them that I would keep it for them if they did not have room for it. I wanted to see what their initial thoughts were.

Their reaction was very touching. They were excited and honored at the thought of having the piano. Being musicians, they recognized the value of the instrument, not to mention the sentimental attachments. Claire recalled her grandmother teaching her to play at that piano and many subsequent hours having fun at that keyboard during her visits with her grandparents.

Before they came, I had sorted out the music that was mine, so I was able to offer to them all the music in the piano bench and all the contents of a trunk of music that Sheila had in the basement. They emptied the contents of both onto my living room floor and spent most of the afternoon being delighted at their finds.

I was very happy for them, but it was a very difficult few hours for me. Sheila didn't really use the music because she didn't need it, but I was watching a review of a lifetime of precious things owned by my favorite musician. I missed her terribly that afternoon and had to work very hard to maintain an appropriate demeanor.

They took measurements of the piano and some photos, gathered up most of the things from the trunk and piano bench, and left with a pledge to let me know what they would do next. They were hopeful that the piano would fit into a spot they had in mind in their little house. I had to feel good about Sheila's prized possession finding a good home. But it was hard.

Over the course of the fall, there were many trips in and out of the house and the relocation of possessions continued gradually. I was a bit surprised by the lack of sentiment, as evidenced by things that nobody wanted: the wedding dishes from their parents' wedding almost fifty years earlier, an afghan that Sheila's mother had made in her favorite color, and candlesticks made by Sheila's dad. I could not throw those things away, so kept them in a safe place until I was better able to make decisions about what to do with them.

By early November, the grandfather clock, mantle clock, and piano were gone. The absence of the clocks made the house quieter. The absence of the piano made me miss Sheila and her music terribly.

And the house was even more of a wreck. Before I began to reconstruct it, I knew I had to deal with Sheila's closet. Her things were in the walk-in closet in the master suite of the house. It was loaded with stuff, and not just her clothes. I briefly sorted through those things and took some for myself. I selected some of her t-shirts, jackets, sweaters and a necklace I had given her.

Then I asked Mark and Tina to come for Sheila's clothes. I was ready for the clothes to be gone and I wanted them to be donated for use by someone else. I just didn't want to be the one to pack those things up. Since they had been offering to help, I brought them into this job.

I mostly stayed out of the closet that day and just left them to do it however they thought best. I didn't want to watch. I could envision all of it dredging up memories of clothes Sheila bought for special occasions or when we were on our trips, or just her favorite things I knew she liked. I was glad for them to take care of that for me. That was another really hard day.

I found that cleaning out her bathroom and her bedside table and her car was excruciating. There were traces of her personality all over the place—her makeup in the bathroom, her hairbrush in her car, her notepad in her bedside table. I had to pace myself. I cried and cried every time I tackled one of these places to clean up. But I kept going. I had to get comfortable in my own house again.

And then there was the dog. Poor Hildey spent long days alone. Even toward the end of Sheila's life, we had the dog in the house because Sheila liked having her there. But when I went back to work, I worked long days. Work was therapeutic for me. It demanded my full attention as I was surrounded by competent and committed people. The hardest part of the work day was coming home to the empty house and missing the time I had spent with Sheila hearing about everything other than a business problem. I had to make different efforts to maintain work/life balance.

My hours were not fair to Hildey. She had no interaction with anyone except for a few hours with me in the evenings. And I was often not in the mood for a high-energy dog. I had promised Sheila that I would look out for Hildey if things didn't turn out well for her. I decided that the best thing for Hildey would be to find her a new home.

I called the dog-sitter, who loved Hildey, and asked for help after explaining my thinking. She validated the decision and promised to help me find a home for her. She asked me to write a little description of Hildey that she could use "You know, to help her find a new forever home. Write it like Hildey is talking. That really works." Right. These dog people really took some getting used to. But if it would help, I was willing. And the two of us agreed to work on finding a home for Hildey.

Ultimately, the dog-sitter had success and just before Thanksgiving, I packed Hildey's stuff in preparation for her to be picked up. I was sure that the decision was right for the dog. I cannot say that I missed her, but the fact that she was gone made me sad because it was another way I had to face the impact of Sheila's death on my life.

Late in the year, my approach to work/life balance took shape when I began to re-paint the house. Everything that was moving out was gone. I moved into the master suite and overtook Sheila's closet with my things. I had my bathroom down the hall remodeled, and replaced the old carpet in the living room. Sheila and I had talked about doing those two things, but had not gotten to them.

I decided to do the painting myself. It was a physical effort, but I could do it at my pace. And I was motivated to get it done to restore my house to be ready for a new future. I painted the dining room first, then the family room, living room and hallway downstairs. Upstairs I painted the hallway, office, three bedrooms, and the little master bath. As I went, I rearranged furniture, hung new pictures, and tried to make it comfortable and welcoming again.

During the final months of 2008, as I adjusted to my new life, I learned that it was not smart to do everything that "Sheila would want me to do" because I could not always predict what she would say or want while she was living. To try to live up to something because I was guessing what she would want seemed like some kind of false idolatry.

I learned that I could not be Sheila. She had so many commendable traits and so many people longed for her presence that I could have tried to assume her roles or befriend her friends. But I realized I couldn't do that. She was gone. We all had to accept that.

I was reminded that I had to do the things I could do and wait until others were not so painful. Christmas was one that had to wait. Sheila loved the tree and the lights of Christmas. She once had me decorating outside when the wind chill was nearly intolerable, a fact that I mentioned to her in subsequent years with some frequency. She looked forward to the baking and cooking and being with her family.

The best I could do in 2008 was to put lights outside. That felt like an appropriate tribute and brightened the house at an otherwise dark time of year. I felt like we needed that, Ernie and me. And I wanted to signal to friends and family that we were doing our best to carry on without Sheila. All was not dark. I was looking to the lights of Christmas.

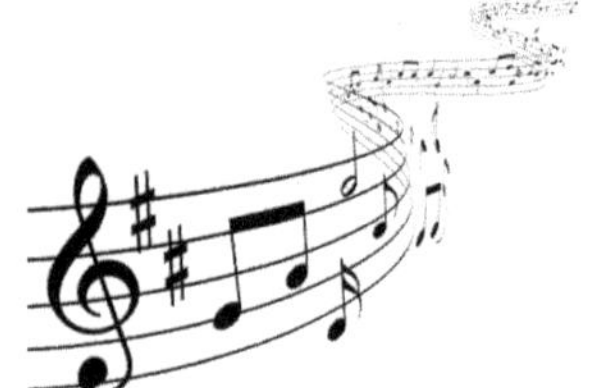

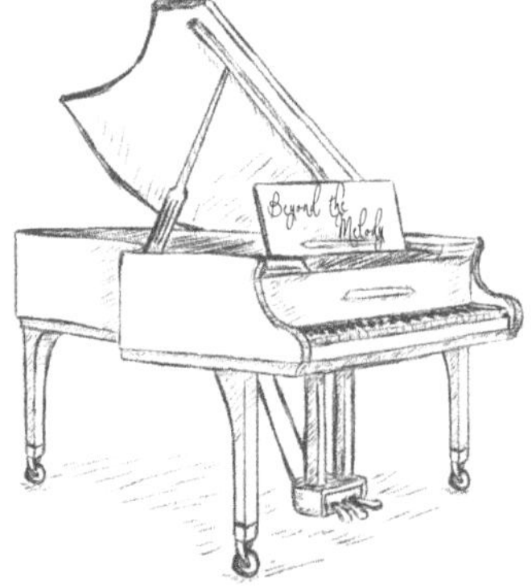
Beyond the Melody

The Melody Lingers On

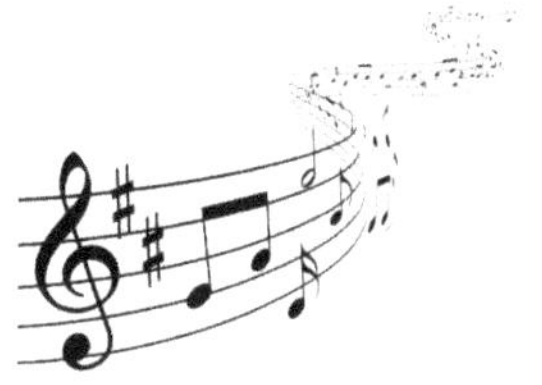

It's been eight years since Sheila died. I retired and returned to Pennsylvania in 2012 to be closer to family and long-time friends. While it was very disruptive and hard to leave my Ohio friends and our house, the one I had lived in the longest in my entire life, I am sure it was another thing I was led to do. And I believed I could thrive afterward, as working through 2008 had reminded me.

Ernie died about a year ago. He was fourteen and the veterinarian called him "elderly" when we were treating his final illness. Several days after he died, it occurred to me that I'm the only one left now from that happy Ohio household. I miss them all—except maybe the dog.

I have many new friends here, some of whom are aware that a person named Sheila was part of my Ohio life. As we get to know each other better and they hear me speak of her so highly, some are asking to learn more. I tell some stories, but they cannot know the extent to which Sheila is still with me. In some ways I've been acting like an extrovert in getting to know my new friends. I sometimes wonder what Sheila would think. I hope she would laugh.

I think the best tribute to another's life is to adopt some of it into your own, to find ways to consciously change yourself to honor what another taught you and meant to you. I try very hard to act with more kindness and generosity toward others.

I am not uncomfortable in hospitals any more. I wipe the handle of the grocery cart every time I go to the store, and I smile when I see dog-walkers clutching their little bags as they stride along past my house, and I still wear that aqua-colored jacket.

Sheila's wedding dishes are in the corner cupboard in my dining room. I have a new chiming clock on the mantle alongside Sheila's dad's candlesticks. As far as I can tell, the clock is in tune. A select "Mrs. Cow" statue is there, too, presiding over the household. I buy tablecloths much more frequently than I ever did before. Sheila's recipe book with the detailed planning notes is in my pantry. I use it regularly. And I make batches of cookies every Christmas season in her memory. I've decorated a Christmas tree and put lights outside every year since I moved here. The lights of Christmas still shine brightly, full of joy.

And as I write, I can see four gorgeous, bright yellow finches hanging from the feeder I refilled just this morning.

Acknowledgments

There is a certain amount of audacity involved when a non-author decides to publish the first book she has ever written. This journey has tested my self-esteem, confidence, and faith. Fortunately, I happen to have good measure of these characteristics, thanks to my parents who have always provided unwavering love and support even when my decisions have caused them concern. Their lives inspire me, form me, and enable me to feel secure no matter what ventures I undertake, as they are models for how to live a faithful life. I would not have had the courage to make the choice to share this writing if they had not provided such a foundation for my life.

I also felt that I needed external validation which was provided by the nine friends who read this book when it was only a typed manuscript in a three-ringed binder. They have continued to be a supportive presence during the preparation of this book and have shown interest in its progress, unstintingly propping me up when I felt unsteady. All are people of intelligence, humor, trustworthiness, and kindness. Their surprising reaction to what I had written emboldened me. Knowing that their friendship is not predicated upon the outcome of publishing is an even greater gift than their interest and input. Most told me that they did not want to be mentioned by name, but I feel compelled to publically acknowledge them, as I would not have written this book without their help.

Regardless of this warm encouragement, I realized I needed some professional guidance. My editor, who has known me since I was sixteen years old, was one of the first to gently encourage me to think about sharing this story. She helped me to become comfortable with the idea, gave me room to struggle with my thoughts and feelings, and waited for me to sort things out in my own mind. Once I was committed, her own experience in writing, editing, and publishing added to my developing confidence. Most of all, her guidance was reassuring and affirming, as it has been for the more than forty years of our friendship. I can't imagine having prepared this story for publication with anyone else.

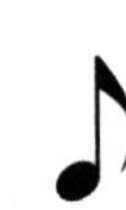

www.ingramcontent.com/pod-product-compliance
Lightning Source LLC
Chambersburg PA
CBHW060745100426
42813CB00032B/3408/J

* 9 7 8 0 9 8 3 7 7 6 8 9 5 *